T0175241

This book has been sponsored by ETHICON Surgical Care, Johnson & Johnson Medical GmbH, Norderstedt, Germany and the European Surgical Institute, Norderstedt, Germany. The authors are responsible for the content of the publication. Information provided in this book is offered in good faith as an educational tool for healthcare professionals. The information has been thoroughly reviewed and is believed to be useful and accurate at the time of its publication, but is offered without warranty of any kind. The authors and the sponsors shall not be responsible for any loss or damage arising from its use. Always refer to the instructions for use that comes with each device for the most current and complete instructions.

Laparoscopic Hysterectomy

Editors

Marc Immenroth
Jürgen Brenner

Authors

Andreas Hackethal
Hans-Rudolf Tinneberg

assisted by

Ellen Markert

Ann-Katrin Bruns, née Güler
Annegret Röhling
Detlev Ruge
Maike Aukstinnis

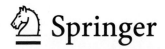
Springer

Authors

Andreas Hackethal, MD, PhD
Senior Gynecologist and Obstetrician
Tagesklinik Altona
Altonaer Str. 59–61
20357 Hamburg, Germany

Hans-Rudolf Tinneberg, MD, PhD
Head of Department of Gynecology and Obstetrics
Universitätsklinikum Gießen
Klinikstr. 32
35392 Gießen, Germany

Editors

Marc Immenroth, PhD
Sales & Business Development Manager Ethicon Surgical Care Germany
Johnson & Johnson MEDICAL GmbH
Robert-Koch-Straße 1
22851 Norderstedt, Germany

Jürgen Brenner, MD
Eric Krauthammer & Dr. Jürgen Brenner
Creative Team-Leadership

ISBN: 978-3-642-38093-8 Laparoscopic Hysterectomy

Bibliografische Information der Deutschen Bibliothek
The Deutsche Bibliothek lists this publication in Deutsche Nationalbibliographie;
detailed bibliographic data are available in the internet at http://dnb.ddb.de.

First published in Germany in 2015 by Springer Berlin Heidelberg
springer.com

SPIN 86252120
Layout and typesetting: Dr. Carl GmbH, Stuttgart, Germany
Printing: Phoenix Print, Würzburg, Germany

18/2122/DK – 5 4 3 2 1 0

EDITORS' PREFACE

This Operation Primer marks the continuation of a series of very successful books, which have gained ever more recognition in recent years. Thanks to consistently positive reviews in renowned specialist publications we are motivated to continue to invest in these "cook books" for surgeons. In response to international demand we plan to release the forthcoming English-language primers in other languages. In addition to the central European languages, Chinese will also be available.

The idea for the Operation Primer series originated in a scientific study entitled "Mental Training in Surgical Education" that formed part of a collaborative project between the surgical department of the University of Cologne, the Institute of Sports and Sports Science of the University of Heidelberg and the European Surgical Institute (ESI) in Norderstedt. The aim of the study was to evaluate the effect of mental training, which has been used successfully in top-class sports for decades, on surgical training. However, in order for mental training to be applied to surgery, it first had to undergo modification. In the course of this modification, the first Operation Primer was produced, the layout of which was largely adopted for the final version presented here. The practice of defining nodal points for operations and then learning these by heart and going through them mentally has been proven to lead to better surgical results. Surgeons approach operations more prepared, are no longer surprised when confronted with the unexpected, and thus operate with more confidence.

The Operation Primers with surgical topics have been updated in this issue by operative intervention in the field of gynecology. The mental training for doctors and the Operation Primer originating from it has gained widespread recognition in the meantime. It was a challenge for us to interest doctors in the mental training and in learning the techniques. One of the important reasons is quite obviously that mental training is not only voluntary, it costs almost nothing. It costs time. You have to get involved to learn the nodal points. Today, the words patient safety have almost become the Word of the Year. A matter of quality. If we ourselves are about to have surgery, we also want to know how to find the best surgeon and that the person who is operating on us can do it really well.

We have only one goal with these guidebooks on nodal points: We want to help improve quality in the operative fields, to facilitate learning and thus to increase patient safety and quality of life.

The renowned gynecological surgeons Prof. Dr. Hans-Rudolf Tinneberg and Dr. Andreas Hackethal PhD have, with their great experience and with dedicated commitment, defined and described the nodal points.

We have also received excellent support from *Dr. Carl GmbH*, which has accompanied us at each stage of the working process and has contributed greatly to making these innovative surgical textbooks what they are. The diagrams, line drawings, etc. were produced mainly by *Thomas Heller*. *Detlev Ruge* was responsible for the pictures featured in this Operation Primer. The existing concept of practical surgical primers has become reality through the publishing company *Springer Medizin Verlag Heidelberg*. Sincere thanks to all of them.

The editors are convinced that the haptic experience of holding a book in one's hand rather than an electronic device has a significant value. You will make a small investment in the book, a bigger one in your time and a large one in your stress management.

"Why not learn from others before we make the mistake ourselves?"

The Editors   May 2015

Hysterectomy for various pathological reasons remains one of the most frequently practiced surgical procedures in gynecology – even with the development of such uterus-sparing procedures as endometrial ablation and high-frequency ultrasound ablation for myomas or intrauterine progestogen-releasing devices.

Nowadays, it is questionable, whether the vaginal hysterectomy can still be considered the "gold standard". The endoscopic techniques, instrumentation and surgeons' skills have advanced steadily over the last several decades. We consider the laparoscopic assisted vaginal hysterectomy (LAVH) a learning procedure on the way to total laparoscopic hysterectomy (TLH). Alternatively, some gynecologists perform laparoscopic supracervical hysterectomies (LASH or LSH). Although the evidence does not point to an advantage for subtotal hysterectomy in preventing prolapse and incontinence, stabilization of the pelvic floor or better sexual functioning, the supracervical hysterectomy is surgically less time-consuming, and intraoperative complication rates are reduced.

From today's perspective, abdominal hysterectomy seems to be an inadequate treatment option for most of the patients and should be reduced to a minimum.

This operation primer summarizes the key steps for the TLH and LSH procedures and indicates possible hazards and complications. Feel free to modify details according to individual needs and preferences!

Our thanks go to Cornelia Wilhelm and Joachim Birkhahn and the OR staff of the Gynecological Department of the Universitätsklinikum Giessen for organizing operating equipment and supporting the photo shooting.

Andreas Hackethal
Hans-Rudolf Tinneberg   May 2015

AUTHORS

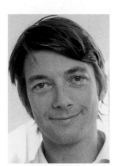

Andreas Hackethal, MD, PhD

– Studied medicine in Kiel, Germany
– 2002 Medical Doctor at Christian-Albrechts-University Kiel, Department of Gynecology
– 2002–2003 Residency at the European Surgical Institute, Norderstedt, Germany
– 2003–2004 Residency at the Department of Gynecology and Obstetrics, Katholisches Marienkrankenhaus Hamburg, Germany
– 2004–2008 Residency at the Department of Gynecology and Obstetrics, Justus-Liebig-University Gießen, Germany
– 2008 Qualified as a gynecologist and an obstetrician
– 2008–2012 Senior Gynecologist and Obstetrician at Justus-Liebig-University Gießen, Germany
– 2012–2014 Fellow in Gynecological Oncology, Queensland Centre of Gynaecological Cancer, Brisbane, Australia
– 2014–2015 Senior Gynecologist and Obstetrician at University Hospital Würzburg, Germany
– Since 2015 Partner Tagesklinik Altona, Hamburg, Germany

Focus of Research and Work
– Clinical instructor at Justus-Liebig-University Gießen
– Regular performance of live procedures in front of audiences worldwide
– Organization of international endoscopy workshops with hands-on training and live surgeries
– Endoscopic treatment of endometrial and cervical cancer
– Endoscopic treatment of deep infiltrating endometriosis (DIE)
– Intra-abdominal adhesions and preventive options
– Objective evaluation of manual skills in endoscopic surgery (with GSES skills lab)

Memberships
– International Society for Gynecological Endoscopy
– European Society for Gynecological Endoscopy
– European Association of Endoscopic Surgery
– European Society of Gynecological Oncology
– German Society for Gynecological Endoscopy (advisory board member since 2007)
– German Society of Gynecology and Obstetrics
– Founder and managing director of the Gießen School of Endoscopic Surgery (GSES) since 2004
– Founder of the Clinical Adhesions, Research and Evaluation Group (CARE-Group) in 2008
– Member of the 'flying doc group', an Ethicon initiative to teach and perform endoscopic surgery within Europe

First author and co-author of numerous articles in journals and books

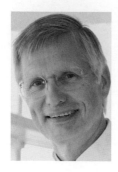

Hans-Rudolf Tinneberg, MD, PhD

– Studied medicine in Kiel, Germany
– 1978 Medical Doctor at Christian-Albrechts-University Kiel, Department of Gynecology
– 1978–1979 Research Scholarship (Australian European Awards Program) Department of Biological Sciences, University of Newcastle, Australia
– 1980–1987 Medical research employee at the Department of Gynecology and Obstetrics, Christian-Albrechts-University Kiel, Germany
– 1986 Qualified as a gynecologist and an obstetrician
– 1987–1992 Senior registrar and lecturer, Head of IVF (in vitro fertilization), Department of Gynecology and Obstetrics, Eberhard-Karls-University Tübingen, Germany
– 1993–2001 Head of Department of Gynecology and Obstetrics, Municipal Hospital Bielefeld-Rosenhöhe, Germany
– 1994–2001 Part-time lecturer, School of Public Health, University Bielefeld, Germany
– Since 2002 Head of Department of Gynecology and Obstetrics, Justus-Liebig-University Gießen, Germany

Focus of Research and Work
– Supervisor of Residency Program, Department of Gynecology and Obstetrics, Justus-Liebig-University Gießen, Germany
– Training courses in endoscopic surgery and reproductive medicine
– Commission member in PhD procedures
– Focus of research: Endometriosis

Memberships
– Executive board member of the International Federation of Fertility Societies
– Executive board member of the International Society of Gynecological Endoscopy
– President of the German Society of Gynecological Endoscopy
– President of the German Society of Reproduction Medicine
– President of the European Endometriosis Information Center
– President of the European Endometriosis League
– Member of the IVF Commission of Medical Chamber Hesse, Germany

First author and co-author of numerous articles in journals and books

Contents

Appendices

Introduction

From an educational point of view, the Operation Primer is somewhat plagiaristic. The layout – and this can be admitted freely – is largely taken over from commonly available cook books. In such books, the ingredients and cooking utensils required to prepare the recipe in question are normally listed first. The most important cooking procedures are then described briefly in the text. Photographs support the written explanations and show what the dish should look like when prepared. Sometimes diagrams and illustrations make individual cooking steps clearer.

Despite these obvious parallels, there is a crucial difference between cook books and the Operation Primer: in the Operation Primer, complicated and complex surgical techniques are described that are intended to help the surgeon and his team perform an operation safely and economically. Ultimately, it always comes down to the patient's welfare. The following must therefore be said early in this introduction:

- The use of the Operation Primer as an aid to operating requires that surgical techniques have first been completely mastered.

- Being alert to possible mistakes is categorically the most important principle when operating; avoiding mistakes is crucial.

As already mentioned in the Editors' preface, the concept of the Operation Primer originated in a scientific study with the title "Mental Training in Surgical Education" that formed part of a collaborative project between the surgical department of the University of Cologne (under Prof. Hans Troidl), the Institute of Sports and Sports Science of the University of Heidelberg, and the European Surgical Institute (ESI) in Norderstedt. Laparoscopic cholecystectomy was the initial focus.

Mental training is derived from top-class sports. This is understood as methodically repeating and consciously imagining actions and movements without actually carrying them out at the same time (cf. Driskell, Copper & Moran, 1994; Feltz & Landers, 1983; Immenroth, 2003; Immenroth, Eberspächer & Hermann, 2008). Scientific involvement with imagining movement has a long tradition in medical and psychological research. As early as 1852, Lotze described how imagining and perceiving movements can lead to a concurrent performance "with quiet movements …" (Lotze, 1852). This phenomenon later became known by the names "Ideomotion" and "Carpenter effect" (Carpenter, 1874).

In the collaborative project, mental training was modified in such a way that it could be employed in the training and further education of young surgeons. In mental training in surgery, surgeons visualize the operation from the inner perspective without performing any actual movements, i.e., they go through the operation step by step in their mind's eye. In the study that was conducted at the ESI, the first Operation Primer was used as the basis for this visualization. In this primer, laparoscopic cholecystectomy was subdivided into individual, clearly depicted steps, the so-called nodal points.

The study evaluated the effect of the mental training on learning laparoscopic cholecystectomy compared with practical training and with a control group. The planning, conduct, and evaluation of the study took seven years (2000–2007), with over 100 surgeons participating.

The results corresponded exactly with the expectations: the mentally trained surgeons improved in a similar degree to those surgeons who received additional practical training on a pelvi trainer simulator (in some subscales even more). Moreover, there was greater improvement in these two groups compared with the control group, which did not receive any additional mental or practical training (cf. in detail, Immenroth, Bürger, Brenner, Nagelschmidt, Eberspächer & Troidl, 2007; Immenroth, Bürger, Brenner, Kemmler, Nagelschmidt, Eberspächer & Troidl, 2005; Immenroth, Eberspächer, Nagelschmidt, Troidl, Bürger, Brenner, Berg, Müller & Kemmler, 2005).

Recently, a significant improvement in surgical knowledge and confidence was shown by both experienced and novice surgeons in another study about mental training in laparoscopic surgery (Arora et al., 2010). Therefore, mental training can be seen as a cost- and time-effective training tool that should be integrated into surgical training.

Furthermore, the study of Immenroth et al. (2007) included a questionnaire to determine the extent to which the mentally trained surgeons accepted mental training as a teaching method in surgery. Mental training was assessed as very positive by all 34 mentally trained surgeons. The Operation Primer received particular acclaim in the evaluation:

• 82 % of the surgeons wished to use similar self-made Operation Primers in their daily work.

• 85 % of the surgeons attributed the success of the mental training at least in part to the Operation Primer.

• 88 % of the surgeons wanted to have these Operation Primers as a fixed component of the course at the ESI.

This positive response to the study was the starting point for the production of the present series of Operation Primers.

Prior to publication, the Operation Primer was developed by methodical and didactical means and then adapted to the readers' needs and wishes. This was carried out following a survey of 93 surgeons (interns, resident doctors, assistant medical directors and medical directors) who participated in surgical courses at the ESI. They evaluated in detail the structure and components by means of a questionnaire.

The results of this survey gave important findings on how to optimize the Operation Primer. The sense and representation of the nodal points, the comprehensibility and detail of the text, and the photographs of the operation were highly valued especially by young surgeons (Güler, Immenroth, Berg, Bürger & Gawad, 2006). The comprehensive research undertaken with this Operation Primer series will ensure its overall value to the reader.

Structure and handling of the Operation Primer

In the present series of Operation Primers, an attempt has been made to standardize the described laparoscopic operations as much as possible. This is achieved first by applying the same format to all operating techniques described. Second, operative sequences that are performed identically in all operations are explained using the same blocks of text as far as possible. By following a general structure for the description of all operations and by using identical text blocks, it was intended to aid recognition of recurring patterns and their translation into action even for different operations.

The Operation Primer is divided into five chapters, each identified by Roman numerals and different register colours on the margin. The contents of the individual chapters will now be explained.

In **Preparations for the operation,** the basic instruments for all laparoscopic operations and then the additional instruments for the specific operation are listed. This is followed by a detailed description of the ENSEAL® device, technology and working principles, the positioning of the patient, attaching the dispersive electrode, skin disinfection, and sterile draping of the patient. A detailed description and an illustration is given of how the operating team is to be positioned. Furthermore, a team time-out checklist is provided as well as a detailed description and an illustration of how to position the transvaginal uterine manipulator. The operative preparation is concluded with emptying the urinary bladder and setting up the equipment.

In the chapter **Creating the pneumoperitoneum – placing the trocar for the scope,** two alternatives are shown in detail: the Veres needle and the trocar with optical obturator. The choice of method is up to the individual surgeon. Both alternatives are employed in surgical practice.

Placing the accessory trocars is explained in detail in the next chapter. The written explanations are supplemented by a diagram. In order to keep a constant overview of the placement of the trocars, even during the following description of the operation sequence, this illustration is shown in diminished size in every single operative step.

The core of the Operation Primer is the chapter **Nodal points.** This is where the actual sequence of the operation is described in detail. However, prior to this detailed explanation, the term nodal point will be explained briefly. In the Editors' preface and introduction, mental training was mentioned as a form of training used successfully in top-class sports for decades, and this is where the term originates. In sports as in surgery, a nodal point is understood as one of those structural components of movement that are absolutely essential for performing the movement optimally. Nodal points have to be passed through in succession and are characterized by a reduction in the degrees of freedom of action. In mental training they act as orientation points for methodical repetition and conscious imagining of the athletic or operative movement (cf. in detail Immenroth et al., 2008).

For every operation in the Operation Primer series, these nodal points were extracted in a prolonged process by the authors in collaboration with the editors. The nodal points represent the basic structural framework of an operation. Because of their particular relevance and for better orientation, all of the nodal points in the Operation Primer are shown on the left on each double page as a flow chart. The current nodal point is highlighted graphically. The instruments required for this nodal point and the specific trocars for it are listed in a box on the right, beside the flow chart.

2 possibilities for creating the pneumoperitoneum: the choice is up to the surgeon

Continuous illustration of the trocar position

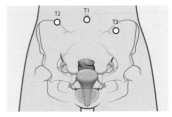

Nodal point = term from top-class sports

Nodal points:
1) absolutely essential
2) successive order
3) no degrees of freedom

Flow chart of the sequence of nodal points on each double page

Maximum of 7±2 instructions per nodal point

Below the instrument box, instructions regarding the nodal point are given as briefly as possible. According to Miller (1956), people can best store 7±2 units of information ("Magical number 7"). Therefore, no more than seven single instructions are listed per nodal point, if possible. With regard to the instructions, it should be noted that the change of instruments between the individual nodal points is not described explicitly as a rule; rather, this is apparent through different instruments in the instrument box.

Watch outs are pointed out in red!

Where necessary, particular moments where special attention is needed are pointed out in red.

Alternatives: In small blue print at the end of the nodal point.

The described operation sequence is only one way of performing the operation safely and economically, namely the way preferred by the authors. Undoubtedly, a number of other equally valid operation sequences exist. As far as possible, notes on alternative methods are given in small blue print at the end of each nodal point.

In the fifth chapter, the **Management of difficult situations and complications** is described in detail. In general, details on adhesions, bleeding, injuries to organs, etc. are given first.

Illustration of anatomical variations, a description of the laparoscopic supracervical hysterectomy (→ p. 62ff), examples of an operation note and details about postoperative management and postoperative complications in the appendices

In the **Appendices** relevant additional surgical procedures and anatomical variations which can occur in the operation sequence and may require a different approach are described first. In order to give the Operation Primer even more practical relevance, an example of an operation note is then reproduced. The appendices also contain helpful hints for the postoperative management, detailed information about postoperative complications and their management, as well as the bibliographical references and an alphabetical index.

(→ p. 35, IV) = reference to chapter IV

In order to avoid repetition, reference is made throughout the text to relevant chapters of the Operation Primer, if necessary. To do this, the Roman numeral of the chapter and the number of the corresponding section are shown in parentheses. Referral is made most often to the fifth chapter, where the management of difficult situations and complications is described. These references are set off in red letters.

All sources in the literature are listed in the bibliography

Finally, it must be pointed out that for better readability of the Operation Primer no bibliographical references at all are given in the text. However, in order to give an overview of the basic and more extensive sources, the entire literature is listed in the bibliography.

Make sure that the following preoperative requirements for laparoscopic hysterectomy have been met:

- The indication for the operation is correct.
- The decision about, whether ovaries without pathology should be removed has been made and the patient was counseled about the benefits of subsequent salpingectomy.
- The patient has given detailed informed written consent.
- The bowel is prepared appropriately prior to laparoscopic surgery.
- Thromboprophylaxis (low-molecular-weight heparin) has been given as per local practice.
- Single-dose perioperative antibiotic prophylaxis has been given.

Basic instruments

- Scalpel with size 11 blade
- 10 ml syringe with size 21 needle for 0.9 % NaCl solution (saline)
- 2 Bullet or Addson forceps
- Open-sided Graves speculum
- Vaginal specula (standard and long)
- Breisky and Haeney retractors
- 2 single tooth tenacula
- Needle holders (short and long, straight and Haeney)
- Suture scissors
- Ring forceps
- Gauze pads
- Swabs with an integral X-ray contrast strip
- Sutures:
    - Fascia: 2–0 absorbable, multifilament (e.g. Vicryl®, Ethicon Products)
    - Subcutaneous: 3–0 absorbable, multifilament or monofilament, as needed
    - Skin: 3–0 absorbable, monofilament or skin adhesive (e. g. Dermabond®, Ethicon Products)

Instruments for the first entry, depending on the type of access:

a) Veres needle (e.g. ENDOPATH® Ultra Veress Insufflation Needle, Ethicon Endo-Surgery)

b) Trocar with optical obturator (e.g. ENDOPATH® XCEL™ bladeless trocar, Ethicon Endo-Surgery)

There should always be a basic laparotomy set in the operating room so that in an emergency a laparotomy can be performed without delay!

Alternative: The usage of antibacterial suture material coated with Triclosan, the Plus Suture generation from Ethicon, is also recommended to reduce the risk of wound infections.

Additional instruments for laparoscopic hysterectomy

- Trocars: (e.g. Endopath XCEL® trocar, Ethicon Endo-Surgery)
  T1: Trocar for the laparoscope (5/7/10–12 mm)
  T2: Accessory trocar (5 mm)
  T3: Accessory trocar (5 mm)
  Additional trocars (5 mm) as needed (T4)

- Angled laparoscope 30° (0° scope, if necessary, for trocar with optical obturator)

- 2 atraumatic grasping forceps (10/12 mm)
- Sealing and transecting device (e.g. ENSEAL® G2 curved or straight tissue sealers)
- Monopolar hook
- Bipolar electrosurgical device
- Berci needle or 5/8 circle needle with small S-retractors (e.g. UR-6 needle with 0 Vicryl®, Ethicon Products)
- Curved Metzenbaum scissors
- Endoscopic needle holders
- Sutures: 2–0 absorbable, monofilament for the vagina
- Suction and irrigation instrument

- Transvaginal uterine manipulator set for culdotomy and vaginal occlusion

Always refer to the instructions for use that come with each device for the most current and complete instructions.

Basic instruments

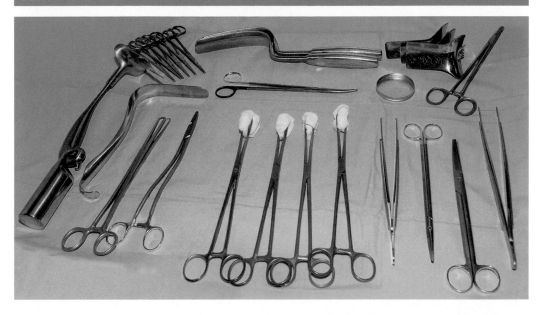

Additional instruments for laparoscopic hysterectomy

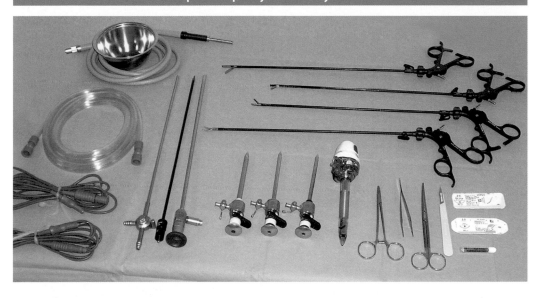

Instrument set: uterine manipulator

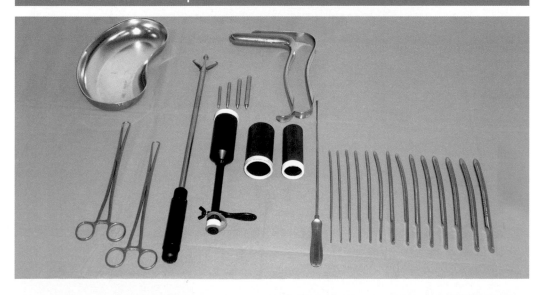

The ENSEAL® device, technology and working principles

Equipment

The ENSEAL® G2 curved or straight tissue sealer is a sterile, single patient use surgical instrument used to coagulate and transect vessels and/or tissue bundles up to and including 7 mm in diameter.

The instrument consists of a grip housing assembly, a rotating shaft, a moveable jaw and an I-BLADE® knife in the jaws.

The instrument shaft can be rotated to facilitate visualization and enable easy access to targeted tissue. The ENSEAL® G2 curved or straight tissue sealer is designed for use exclusively with the Generator G11 (GEN11). The entire ENSEAL® G2 curved or straight tissue sealer line with curved and straight devices in multiple 5 mm shaft lengths is designed for superior tissue sealing by providing uniform compression, controlling temperature and minimizing thermal spread.

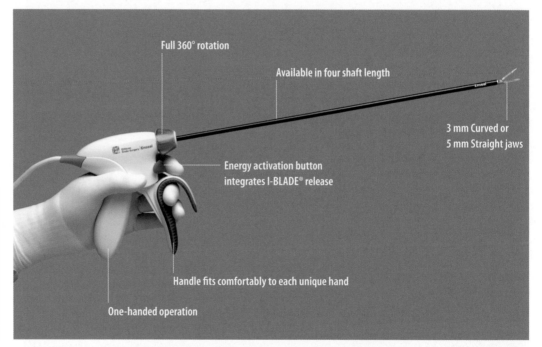

Full 360° rotation

Available in four shaft length

3 mm Curved or
5 mm Straight jaws

Energy activation button
integrates I-BLADE® release

Handle fits comfortably to each unique hand

One-handed operation

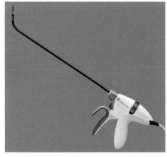

ENSEAL® G2 articulating tissue sealer

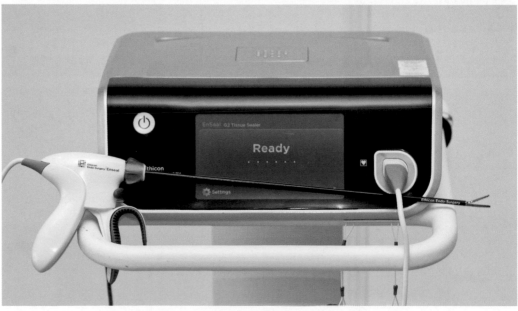

ETHICON generator GEN11 for ENSEAL® and HARMONIC® technology

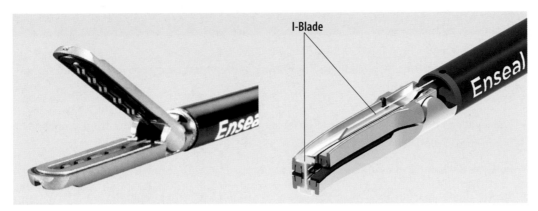

I-Blade

ENSEAL jaws with positive temperature coefficient (PTC)   **ENSEAL jaws with I-BLADE®**

The ENSEAL® technology

The exclusive ENSEAL® technology differs from other bipolar instruments to provide superior sealing. Its patented I-BLADE® forces the jaws of the device together as it advances, resulting in high uniform compression along the entire length of the jaws.

The temperature regulating positive temperature coefficient (PTC) material in the ENSEAL® devices is designed to minimize sticking. A polymer compound within the jaw uses PTC technology to keep temperature at about 100°C. When tissue temperature is below 100°C, conductive chains of molecules permit energy delivery. Above 100°C, the chains break apart, automatically interrupting energy and limiting temperature increase.

The ENSEAL® offset electrode configuration is designed to minimize thermal spread. The ENSEAL® offset electrode configuration surrounds the active electrode with multiple return electrodes. This design helps contain current flow within the device jaws.

The ENSEAL® working principles

Step 1: Connect the instrument power cord to the generator (GEN 11).

Step 2: Position targeted tissue within open jaws.

Step 3: Close jaws around the tissue by gently squeezing the closing handle to the first mechanical stop.

Step 4: Press the energy activation button to activate energy and unlock the I-BLADE® knife. The generator provides audible feedback (Tone 1) as energy is delivered to the grasped tissue.

Step 5: Continue squeezing the closing handle to gradually advance the I-BLADE® knife. The generator tone changes to an increased pitch (Tone 2) when the tissue impedance threshold is reached and the I-BLADE® knife is ready to be fully advanced.

Step 6: Complete the firing cycle by ensuring the closing handle is squeezed to the fully closed position and stops against the grip housing.
Once the I-BLADE® is fully advanced and the tissue impedance threshold has been reached, the generator provides one short beep (Tone 3) that indicates the cycle is complete and automatically stops delivery of energy.

Step 7: Release the closing handle and the energy activation button.

This information does not replace the instructions for use provided with each instrument.

Positioning of the patient

The technical fittings, especially the operating table, must be approved and functional for the patient's weight!

- Use a padded board or foam mattress as table surface to prevent the patient from sliding when put in steep Trendelenburg.

- Position the patient in modified dorsal lithotomy position with feet flatly supported.

- Stretch thighs apart to allow vaginal access and position legs with a slight flexure.

- Arms should be wrapped close to the patient's body with the hands and arms adducted.

- Pad elbow to avoid compression injury.

- Maintain in unaltered supine position and drop table to lowest height before insufflation.

- After creating the pneumoperitoneum and inserting the primary trocar for the laparoscope tilt the patient into Trendelenburg position (i.e., head down 30–40°) as much as tolerated.

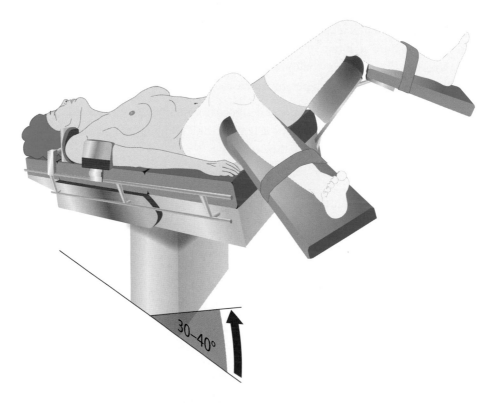

Dispersive electrode

- Before applying the dispersive electrode over the outer thigh, ensure that the skin at this site and areas in contact with the table are absolutely dry.

- Stick the entire surface of the electrode carefully above the greatest possible muscle mass (e.g. on the upper thigh). The conducting cable must be at the greatest possible distance from the operating field.

When using monopolar current, always guard against burns on moist areas of the skin due to aberrantly conducted current!

Skin disinfection

- Disinfect the lower buttocks, vulva, and vagina.

- Disinfect the abdominal skin from the costal arch to the pubic symphysis.

- Pay particular attention to mechanical clearing and disinfection of the umbilicus.

- Pay particular attention to careful disinfection of all skin folds.

Sterile draping

- Lay sterile drapes on the table under the buttock region and cover both legs.

- Drape the operating field for laparoscopy with sterile drapes so that the area is limited cranially at the level of the xiphoid, just above the pubic symphysis caudally, and by the midaxillary lines laterally.

Positioning of the operating team

- The surgeon stands to the left or right at the level of the patient's abdomen.

- The camera assistant stands to the right or left at the level of the patient's abdomen.

- The scrub nurse stands on the same side as the surgeon at the level of the patient's lower leg.

- The assistant moving the uterine manipulator sits between the patient's spread legs.

- Two monitors are located, one in the line of vision of the surgeon and one in the camera assistant's.

Alternative: If only one monitor is available, locate it between the patient's legs.

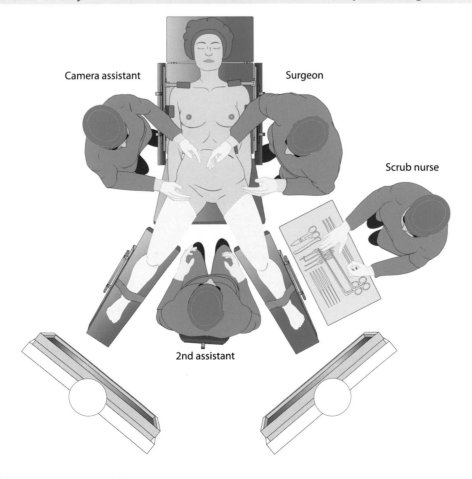

Team time-out

Minimizing patients' risks is a major issue for every surgeon. Besides its relevance for the individual patient, the hospital-wide safety culture is also an important indicator of treatment quality.

Promoted mainly by the World Health Organization (WHO) project "Safe Surgery Saves Lives", checklists have been developed to improve patient safety. Wrong-site surgery is avoided by a review done directly before the start of the operation. These checklists have been introduced into clinical routine with the so-called team time-out.

Basically, this time-out is intended to give the whole team in the operating room the opportunity to re-check all important safety aspects.

The checklists provided by the WHO should be adapted for the individual setting by each surgical department and should be integrated into the already existing safety efforts. However, it is very important that every member of the team understands that "team time-out" is not additional and needless paperwork but rather a necessary tool to reduce the number of adverse events in the operating room by strengthening the collaboration among operating room personnel.

To minimize patients' risks, re-check together with the whole team in the operating room all important safety aspects using the following checklist:

Prior to the operation:

☐ All members of the operating team have been introduced (anesthetist, surgeon, scrub nurses) and are known.
☐ Identity of the patient has been checked by the anesthetist, the surgeon and the nursing staff using the patient's chart and the patient's bracelet and, if possible, by asking the patient personally.
☐ Existence of a valid written, informed consent of the patient to anesthesia and operation has been reviewed.
☐ Planned operation, side and height localization, as well as positioning of the patient, fit with the documented diagnosis.
☐ The patient has been positioned correctly.
☐ All necessary instruments are available.
☐ The required imaging is available.
☐ Relevant medication, especially single-dose perioperative antibiotic prophylaxis, has been given.

Before patient leaves operating room:

☐ Counts of instruments, cloths, compresses etc. are correct and complete.
☐ The specimens for pathology are labeled correctly and have been passed on to the pathologist.
☐ Any equipment failure has been reported to the sterilization or engineering department.
☐ Quality of supplies in the appropriate further processing unit is verified.
☐ The postoperative prescription chart is filled in and is carried along with the patient.

Positioning of a transvaginal uterine manipulator

1. Insert open-sided Graves speculum.

2. Grasp anterior cervix with single tooth tenaculum.

3. Remove Graves speculum.

4. Insert short or long weighted vaginal speculum.

5. Place cervix on downward traction with tenaculum.

6. Probe and dilate internal os to required diameter.

7. Introduce and set the uterine manipulator.

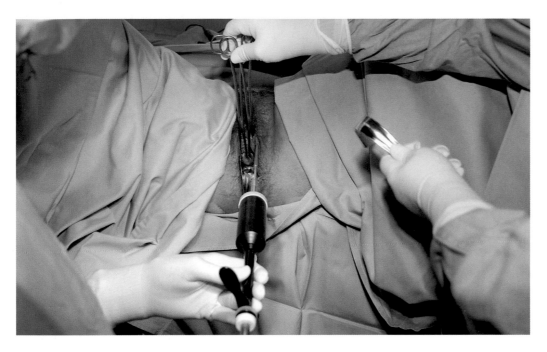

Uterine manipulator prior to introduction

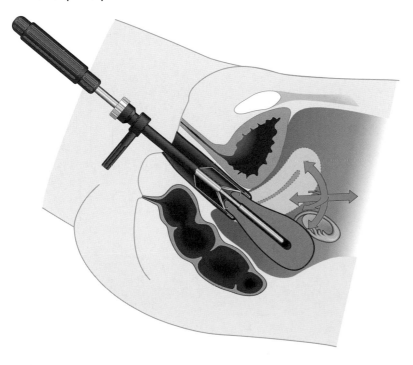

Uterine manipulator allowing a three-dimensional mobilization of the uterus.

Emptying the urinary bladder

- In order to reduce the risk of urinary bladder injuries, make sure that the patient's bladder is emptied preoperatively by placing a temporary transurethral catheter.

Setting up the equipment

- Turn on the generator for any electrosurgical and vessel sealing device and ensure that the default or manual settings are appropriate for the intended use.

- Position the foot pedal within comfortable range of the operating surgeon.

- Set-up and attach the suction-irrigation device.

- Attach smoke evacuation tubing to accessory trocar (of largest dimension).

CREATING THE PNEUMOPERITONEUM – PLACING THE TROCAR FOR THE SCOPE

There are two ways of creating a pneumoperitoneum commonly used in gynecology:

a) Veres needle (closed technique)

b) Trocar with optical obturator

Because of the large variety of trocars available and the resulting variety of methods of introducing the trocars, follow their individual instruction manuals!

a) Veres needle (closed technique)

Blind insertion of the Veres needle or primary trocar creates the greatest risk during laparoscopy, including damage to the viscera and all of the underlying retroperitoneal vessels.

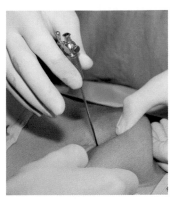

Insertion of the Veres needle

> Size 11 scalpel
> Veres needle
> 10 ml syringe with NaCl solution
> Trocar for the laparoscope T1 (5/7/10–12 mm)

Incise the umbilicus.

Carefully insert the Veres needle vertically with hand supported above the skin incision. The penetration of the abdominal wall layers by the Veres needle can be felt or even heard.

When inserting the Veres needle, take care
• to go in perpendicular to the abdominal wall (→ p. 58, V-4a),
• to support the hand holding the needle, and
• not to use excessive force in order to avoid blood vessel and organ injuries in the event of loss of resistance (→ p. 57, V-2; V-3)!

Check the correct position of the Veres needle by applying the following obligatory safety tests (also known as "Semm tests"):

Aspiration test
Attach a 10 ml syringe filled with NaCl solution to the Veres needle. It should be possible to aspirate air as a sign that the intra-abdominal position is correct. The aspiration of free blood or liquid stool requires immediate attention.

Injection test
Inject NaCl solution through the Veres needle into the abdominal cavity. This can be done easily if it is in the correct position. Increased resistance of the syringe plunger indicates a possible incorrect position of the Veres needle.

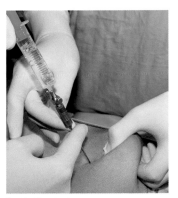

Aspiration test

Alternative: When using the Endopath® Veress Needle Ultra (Ethicon Endo-Surgery), the valve is opened to perform the injection test, whereupon the NaCl solution is released into the abdominal cavity if the Veres needle is in the correct position. In addition, the red marker ball drops down, indicating that NaCl solution is released into the abdominal cavity.

CREATING THE PNEUMOPERITONEUM

Slurp test

Apply one drop of NaCl solution onto the cone of the Veres needle, placing it convex on the opening. Now pull up the abdominal wall, making sure not to fix the Veres needle with your hand. Elevating the abdominal wall will create a partial vacuum, which in turn will cause the drop of NaCl to be sucked into the abdominal cavity, provided the Veres needle is correctly placed. A substantial vacuum will cause an additional "slurping" sound to be heard at the cone of the Veres needle.

If the safety tests indicate that the Veres needle has been placed correctly, attach the gas supply tubing.

Opening pressure should be less than 8 mmHg.

Higher intra-abdominal resting pressure or no flow may indicate that the tip of the Veres needle is obstructed, e.g. by the greater omentum (→ **p. 57, V-3a**). In this case, perform the following test:

Manometer test

In order to release the Veres needle, manually lift up the abdominal wall. This should result in an obvious pressure drop. If this is not the case, remove the Veres needle, inspect the tip for intestinal content, and then place it again.

Insufflate the CO_2 until the preselected maximum pressure of 20 mmHg is reached. Clinical signs of adequate insufflation include loss of liver dullness followed by symmetric expansion and tympany of the abdominal wall.

> **To be sure that the Veres needle has been placed correctly, check for an adequate flow during the CO_2 insufflation (2.5 to 3 l/min) and an appropriate increase in pressure on the insufflator!**

Remove the Veres needle from the skin incision and inspect the tip for intestinal content.

Now place the primary trocar for the laparoscope in the skin incision. To do so use either

• a trocar with a blunt tip (5/7/10–12 mm) or

• a trocar with optical obturator (5/7/10–12 mm).

> **When inserting the trocar, take care**
> • **to go in perpendicular to the abdominal wall,**
> • **to support the trocar with the hand, and**
> • **not to use excessive force in order to avoid blood vessel and organ injuries in the event of loss of resistance (→ p. 57, V-2; V-3)!**

Secure the gas tubing to the trocar, reconfirm the intra-abdominal position, and reduce the pressure to 15 mmHg after placing all of the accessory trocars.

b) Trocar with optical obturator

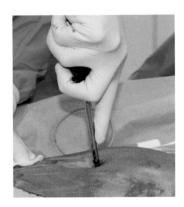

Size 11 scalpel
Trocar (5/7/10–12 mm) with optical obturator
Laparoscope (0°)

Incise the umbilicus (as in closed technique).

> Be careful with extremely slim patients. Incise superficially in order to avoid bowel or vascular injury.

> Ensure that the skin incision is the correct diameter:
> - An incision that is too small can make the insertion of the trocar much more difficult. Inadvertent organ injury may result once the skin is passed from applying excessive force on the trocar. Check the girth of the incision by placing the trocar into its base while untracted.
> - An incision that is too large can result in gas loss and trocar dislocation (→ p. 58, V-4b)!

Insert the laparoscope into the optical obturator located in the trocar and lock into place.

Place the transparent conical tip into the umbilical incision. Now carefully push the different layers of the abdominal wall tangentially apart by applying light pressure and using to-and-fro rotating movements of the blunt obturator tip. The special construction of the obturator allows the layers to be identified before they are pushed apart.

Perform this tissue separation and the final perforation of the peritoneum under constant vision.

> When inserting the trocar, take care
> - to go in perpendicular to the abdominal wall,
> - to support the trocar with the hand, and
> - not to use excessive force in order to avoid blood vessel and organ injuries in the event of loss of resistance (→ p. 57, V-2; V-3)!

Finally, remove the laparoscope together with the obturator from the trocar.

Secure the gas tubing to the trocar, reconfirm the intra-abdominal position, and reduce the pressure from 20 to 15 mmHg after placing all of the accessory trocars.

> **T1:** Trocar for the laparoscope (5/7/10–12 mm)
> **T2:** Accessory trocar (5 mm)
> **T3:** Accessory trocar (5 mm)
> Additional trocars (5 mm) as needed
> Size 11 scalpel

Insert the laparoscope into the trocar (T1).

Explore the abdominal cavity to assess for any pathological changes and to identify any injuries that could change the surgical strategy or even prevent continuation of the operation (→ **p. 57, V-2; V-3**). Place the patient in steep Trendelenburg position.

Once the location, configuration, and size of the uterus have been ascertained, selectively place the accessory trocars T2 and T3 on both sides caudally and laterally from the umbilicus. Palpate the anterior iliac spines as anatomical reference points. Choose the accessory trocar sites and use transillumination to prevent injury to major cutaneous vessels including the superficial epigastric vessels as each accessory trocar is inserted under direct vision (→ **p.57, V-1; V-2**).

Moreover, carefully identify the inferior epigastric vessels to avoid injury as they course cephalo-caudally between the medial umbilical ligament and exit of the round ligament.

Incise the skin superficially with a scalpel to approximate the intended trocar diameter, and then superficially widen to 5–7 mm. The accessory trocars are then sequentially inserted through the abdominal wall under direct vision.

> When placing an accessory trocar, make sure that
> • each skin incision is adequate incised to accommodate the outer diameter
> • the trocar is inserted under direct vision to avoid injury (→ p. 57, V-2; V-3),
> • the direction of entry is angled towards the uterus once the tip of the trocar has traversed the peritoneum
> • the trocar is directed towards the pelvis, as subsequent correction will be difficult, especially in obese patients.

A midline suprapubic trocar, positioned at the height of the fundus of the uterus can be useful for larger fibroids.

> There are many methods for determining the location of the accessory trocars. While the following placements are the authors' preference, the ultimate arrangement should suit the individual needs of each surgeon.

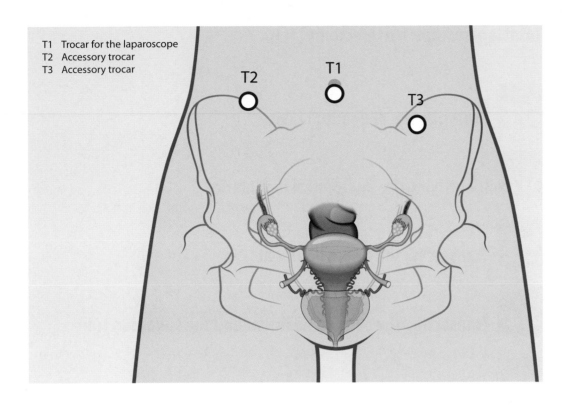

T1 Trocar for the laparoscope
T2 Accessory trocar
T3 Accessory trocar

Total laparoscopic hysterectomy (TLH)

01 Exploring the abdominal cavity

02 Identifying the anatomical landmarks

03 Transecting the round ligament

04 Transecting the ovarian ligament and the Fallopian tube

05 Dissecting the broad ligament

06 Identifying the ureter

07 Exposing and sealing the uterine vessels

08 Skeletonizing the cervix

09 Resecting the uterus

10 Closing the vaginal cuff

11 Finishing the operation

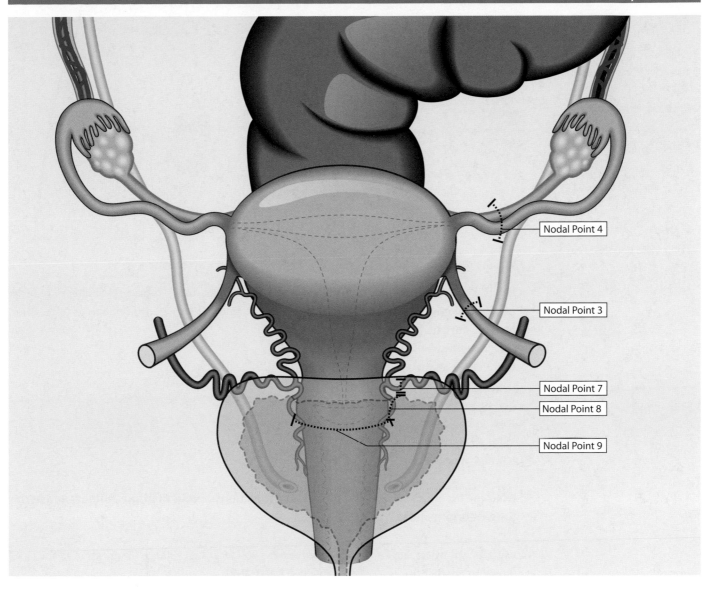

Nodal Point 4

Nodal Point 3

Nodal Point 7

Nodal Point 8

Nodal Point 9

NODAL POINTS

1 Exploring the abdominal cavity

T1   Laparoscope
T2   Atraumatic grasping forceps
T3   Atraumatic grasping forceps

– Curved Metzenbaum scissors as needed

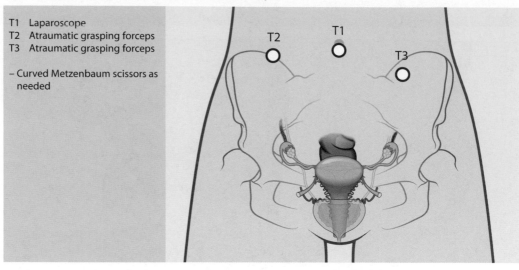

Examine the abdominal cavity carefully by inspecting it in a systematic way.

- Pelvis: Peritoneum of dome of the bladder, round ligament, tubes, ovaries, peritoneum of ovarian fossa, uterosacral ligaments, Pouch of Douglas, internal hernial orifices, uterus (size, color, possible deviation)
- Cecum with appendix
- Right upper abdomen: liver and gallbladder
- Greater omentum
- Left upper abdomen: stomach
- Descending colon
- Sigmoid colon
- Jejunum and ileum

> **Examine for adhesions, erythema, vascular injections, serous fluid, pus, tumors and peritoneal abnormalities.**

Evaluate each trocar site for significant adhesions and bleeding. Change the position of the laparoscope to another trocar if necessary (→ **p. 57, V-1; V-2**).

Lyze any significant adhesions to sufficiently reestablish normal anatomy using sharp dissection with or without coagulation.

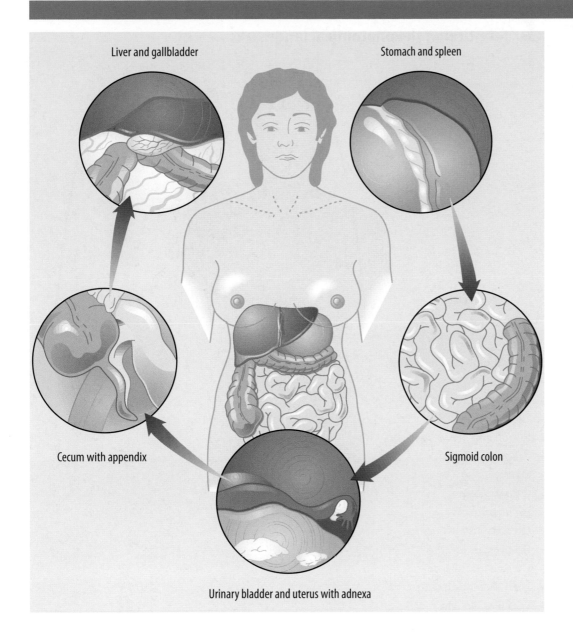

Liver and gallbladder

Stomach and spleen

Cecum with appendix

Sigmoid colon

Urinary bladder and uterus with adnexa

2 Identifying the anatomical landmarks

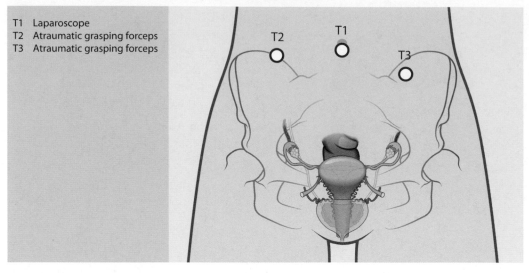

T1   Laparoscope
T2   Atraumatic grasping forceps
T3   Atraumatic grasping forceps

Systematically identify the following anatomical landmarks:

- Medial umbilical ligament
- Bladder
- Vesico-uterine fold
- Uterus
- Round and broad ligaments
- Fallopian tubes
- Ovaries
- Ovarian fossae
- Pelvic brim
- Ureters
- Iliac vessels
- Uterine vasculature
- Uterosacral ligaments
- Pouch of Douglas
- Rectum
- Aorta

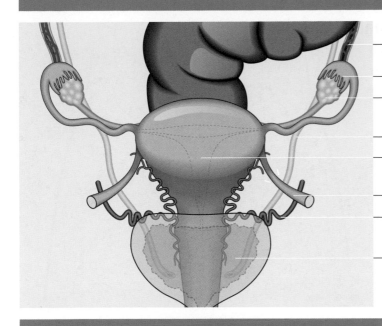

Infundibulopelvic ligament

Fallopian tube

Ovary

Ureter

Uterus

Round ligament

Uterine artery

Urinary bladder

Round ligament and left ovary

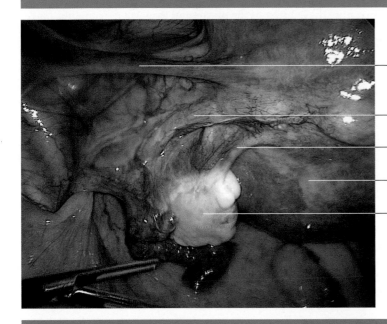

Round ligament

Fallopian tube (discontinued in former sterilization)

Infundibulopelvic ligament

Uterus

Ovary

Entering the pouch of Douglas

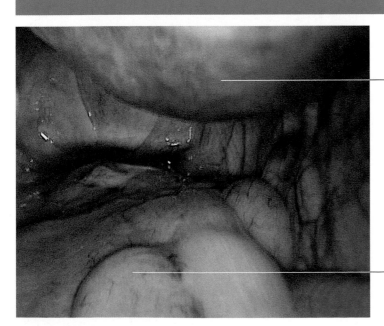

Uterus

Rectum

3 Transecting the round ligament

T1 Laparoscope
T2 ENSEAL® G2 Curved & Straight Tissue Sealers (or T3)
T3 Atraumatic grasping forceps (or T2)

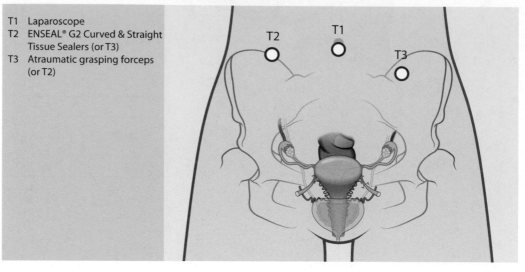

Push the manipulator cranially and to the patient's right side to provide maximal visualization and access before dissecting and separating the left part of the uterus and associated ligaments.

Grasp the left round ligament laterally with an atraumatic forceps.

Insert the ENSEAL® device and place the jaws around the mid-portion of the round ligament about 4–5 cm lateral to the uterus.

Please find detailed information on the ENSEAL® working principles on (→ **p. 21, I**).

Then seal and transect the round ligament to enter and separate the anterior and posterior leaves of the broad ligament.

To achieve reliable hemostasis and efficient ligation with ENSEAL®, slowly advance the I-BLADE® by simultaneously activating energy.

> **Avoid dissection close to the uterine wall where the ascending uterine vessels and numerous small veins are located (the risks of active and back bleeding) (→ p. 57, V-2).**

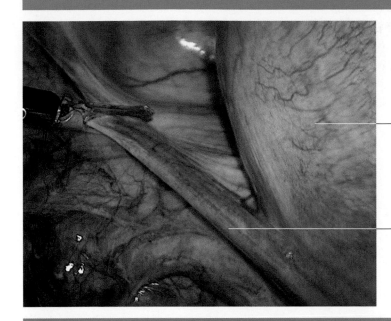

Uterus

Round ligament

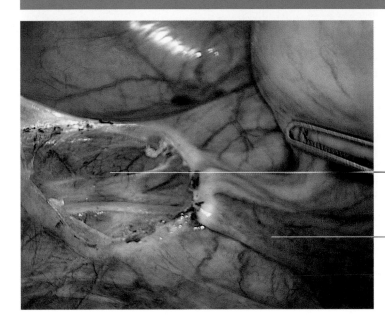

Posterior leaf of broad ligament

Round ligament (stump)

NODAL POINTS

4 Transecting the ovarian ligament and the Fallopian tube

T1   Laparoscope
T2   ENSEAL® G2 Curved & Straight Tissue Sealers (or T3)
T3   Atraumatic grasping forceps (or T2)

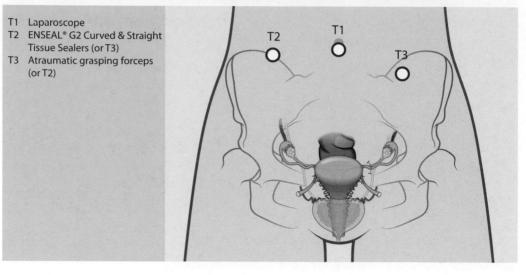

If salpingo-oophorectomy is considered, open broad ligament and identify ureter prior to dissection of infundibulopelvic ligament (→ p. 70 Appendices).

If patient was counseled for salpingectomy with ovarian conservation, transect the mesosalpinx and keep the tube attached to the uterus.

Grasp the left tubo-ovarian pedicle with an atraumatic forceps near the uterus (approximately 1 to 1.5 cm from the uterine wall).

Seal and transect the left ovarian ligament and the left Fallopian tube.

Be careful not to dissect too close to the uterine wall.

Avoid dissection close to the uterine wall where the ascending uterine vessels and numerous small veins are located (the risks of active and back bleeding) (→ p. 57, V-2).

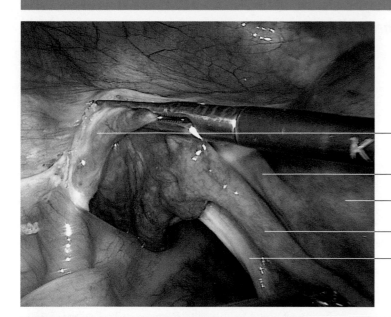

Infundibulopelvic ligament

Round ligament

Uterus

Fallopian tube

Ovarian ligament

Ovarian ligament and Fallopian tube transected

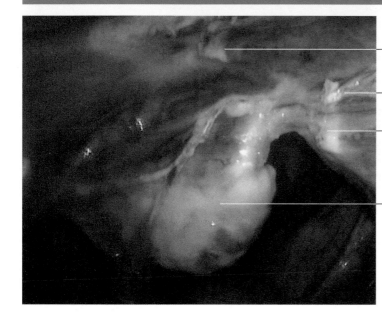

Round ligament (stump)

Fallopian tube (stump)

Ovarian ligament (stump)

Ovary

5 Dissecting the broad ligament

T1 Laparoscope
T2 ENSEAL® G2 Curved & Straight Tissue Sealers (or T3)
T3 Atraumatic grasping forceps (or T2)

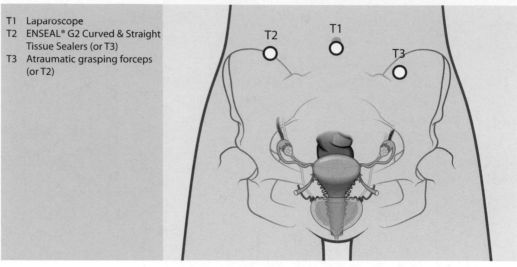

Grasp the lateral broad ligament with an atraumatic forceps.

Mechanically separate the anterior and posterior leaves of the broad ligament. Dissect caudally in a curvilinear fashion toward the isthmus by sealing and cutting as described above (NP 3). Avoid lateral dissection to avoid retroperitoneal bleeding.

Alternative: The uterine vessels including the pelvic ureter may be clarified by dissecting into the broad ligament caudally and laterally.

Identify the left ureter by observing its peristalsis along the lateral pelvic sidewall (NP 6).

Dissect delicately and methodically, and utilize prophylactic and targeted desiccation to minimize inadvertent injury, bleeding, and staining of otherwise clarified tissues.

Be careful while dissecting the broad ligament to minimize inadvertent injury.

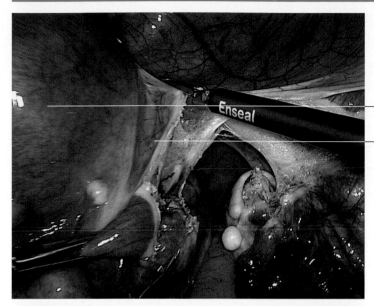

Uterus

Broad ligament

Continuing separation

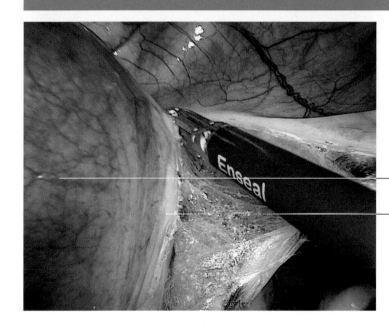

Uterus

Broad ligament

6 Identifying the ureter

T1   Laparoscope
T2   ENSEAL® G2 Curved & Straight Tissue Sealers (or T3)
T3   Atraumatic grasping forceps (or T2)

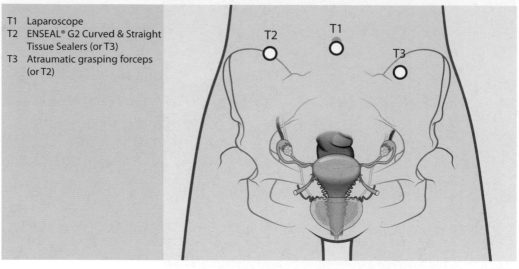

Identify the course of the ureter before continuing to dissect the parametrium.

Preferentially use a blunt instrument to provoke peristalsis. The ureter is best identified where it passes over the left pelvic brim, just medial to the infundibulopelvic vessels. From here it can be visualized or dissected as it travels into the cardinal ligament and then into the posterior bladder close to the vaginal fornix.

Provoke peristalsis with a blunt instrument to identify the course of the ureter before further dissecting the parametrium.

Alternative: Since the ureter and parietal peritoneum are intrinsically attached, displace it laterally by making a linear relaxing incision into the peritoneum medially and then pushing the uterus cranially.

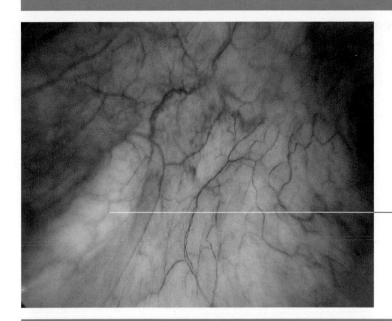

Left ureter (seen through the peritoneal membrane)

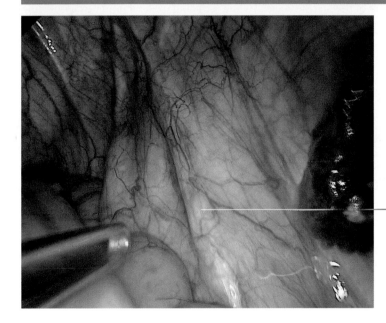

Right ureter

7 Exposing and sealing the uterine vessels

T1   Laparoscope
T2   Atraumatic grasping forceps (or T3)
T3   ENSEAL® G2 Curved & Straight Tissue Sealers (or T2)

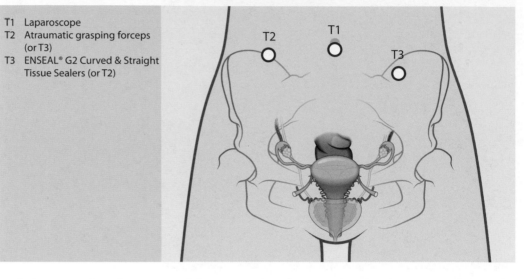

Push the uterus strongly in a cranial direction and to the patient's right. These manipulations will facilitate access to and exposure of the uterine vessels, while reducing ureteral injury by displacing this structure lateral to the dissection.

Continue to divide the anterior leaf of the broad ligament down and then across the isthmus, keeping the dissection caudal to the vesicouterine fold. Dissect until the pubocervical fascia is clarified in order to separate the bladder downward to the level of the anterior vaginal fornix using sharp and blunt dissection.

Continue dissecting the posterior leaf of the broad ligament caudally and medially to the uterosacral ligament and identify the uterine vessels. Identification is sufficient when the fascia of the pericervical ring has been clarified both anterior and posterior to the uterine vessels.

Keep the uterus on cranial traction and take care to avoid marked anterior or posterior rotation. Sequentially grasp, seal and transect the uterine vessels.

Perform nodal points 3–7 on the opposite side.

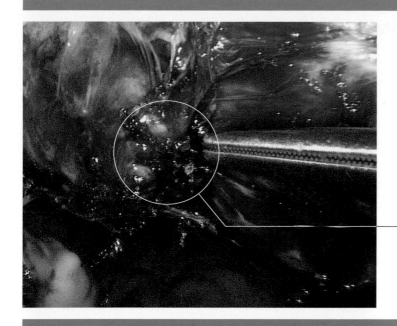

Vascular stump (uterine artery)

Vascular stump (right side)

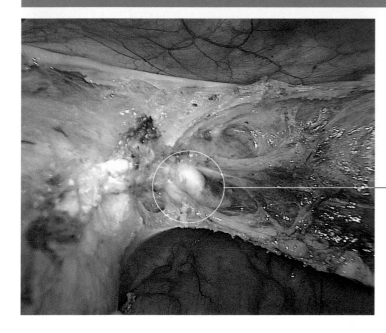

Vascular stump (uterine artery)

8 Skeletonizing the cervix

T1 Laparoscope
T2 ENSEAL® G2 Curved & Straight Tissue Sealers (or T3)
T3 Atraumatic grasping forceps or tenaculum as needed (or T2)

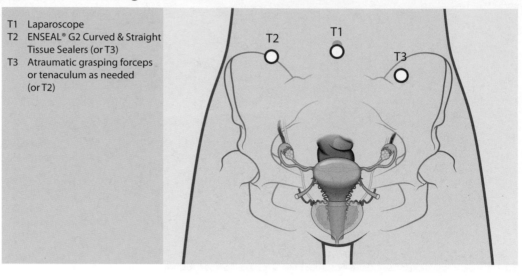

Slip the vaginal delineating tube with a ceramic ring on its top over the manipulator shaft into the vagina. Push the manipulator cranially and move it to the patient's right side. (In case of a different set-up, please refer to the manipulator's manual.)

Ensure that the anterior dissection has sufficiently mobilized the bladder of the cervix to the level of the anterior vaginal fornix.

Move the uterus ventrally using the manipulator and/or a tenaculum (T2 or T3) to dissect the posterior peritoneum between the uterosacral ligaments, considering a preservation of these structures.

Consider preserving the uterosacral ligaments.

Leaving the uterosacral ligaments intact and incorporating them into the vaginal suture may help to stabilize the integrity of the pelvic floor.

Vesicouterine peritoneal fold

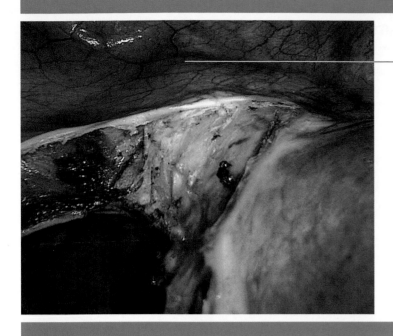

Vesicouterine peritoneal fold

Skeletonizing the cervix

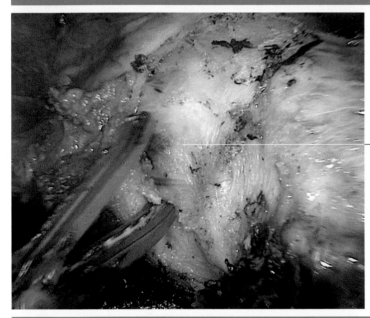

Cervix uteri: pericervical ring

Dissecting cranially from uterosacral ligaments

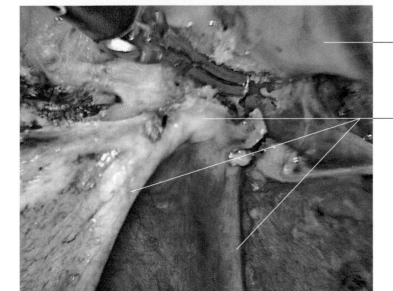

Uterus

Uterosacral ligaments

9 Resecting the uterus

T1   Laparoscope
T2   Monopolar hook (or T3)
T3   Atraumatic grasping forceps
       (or T2)

– Bipolar electrosurgical device
– Suction and irrigation
   instrument

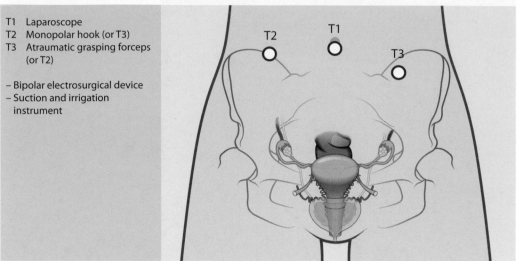

Continue to push the uterus linearly in a cranial direction using the uterine manipulator. Identify the ceramic ring of the manipulator by the resultant bulge and/or by palpation with a blunt instrument. The tension induced by the manipulator allows for an accurate culdotomy incision into the anterior vaginal fornix. Take care to avoid a marked twist with the manipulator, which may cause unintentional entry into the lateral vaginal fornix.

Begin the culdotomy at the anterior fornix using the chosen energy modality. Continue the culdotomy from the posterior fornix after anteflecting the uterus, and preserve the pericervical ring. Join the anterior cut alongside the ceramic ring of the manipulator. Ensure that the cardinal ligaments on each side are incised medial to each uterine artery pedicle. Keep the manipulator pushed cranially with moderate force. Stretching the vaginal fornices cranially further distances the incision line from the bladder and the ureter while enhancing visibility.

> **Begin the culdotomy at the anterior fornix. Continue the culdotomy from the posterior fornix and join the incision circumferentially. Stretch the vaginal fornices by keeping the manipulator pushed cranially.**

Whereas most bleeding along the vaginal cuff will be controlled by suturing, brisk bleeders can be controlled by bipolar electrosurgery using episodic contact desiccation to minimize delayed thermal necrosis.

On completion, remove the resected uterus by pulling downward into the vagina using the transvaginal uterine manipulator. Detach the manipulator and leave the fundus in the vagina to occlude and maintain the pneumoperitoneum.

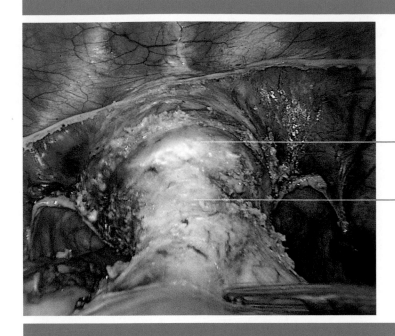

Ceramic ring identifiable in the upper vagina

Cervix uteri skeletonized

Resecting the uterus

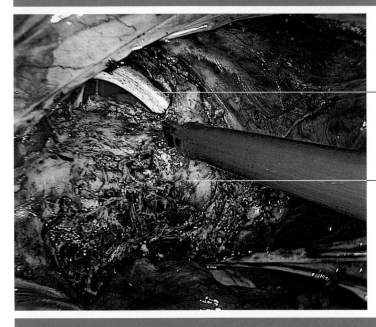

Ceramic ring of the manipulator

Cervix uteri

Resected uterus, held by manipulator

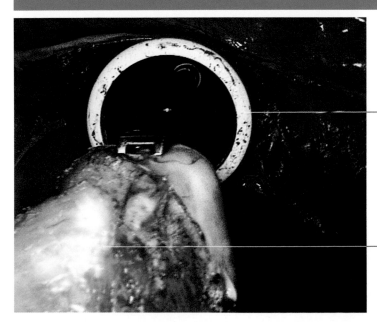

Ceramic ring

Resected uterus

10 Closing the vaginal cuff

T1 Laparoscope
T2 Endoscopic needle holder
T3 Endoscopic needle holder

Sutures:
– Vaginal cuff suture: 2–0
  absorbable monofilament

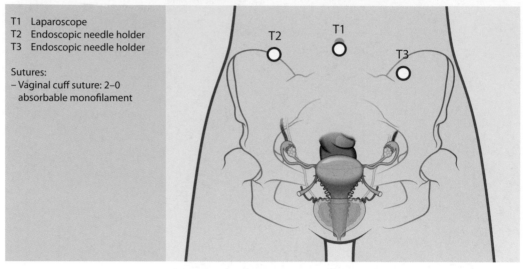

Either use the extirpated uterus or place the tube of the manipulator in the vaginal cuff to maintain the pneumoperitoneum and to help position the margins of the vaginal cuff.

Insert a needle holder with 2–0 absorbable monofilament thread in approximately 20 cm length.

Start with one vaginal corner and continuously suture the vaginal cuff. To help reduce the risk of postoperative vaginal dehiscence, close the culdotomy either with interrupted mattress stitches or in two consecutive layers using full thickness bites with a non-reactive absorbable suture (e.g. PDS®).

Alternative: Suture the vaginal cuff transvaginally.

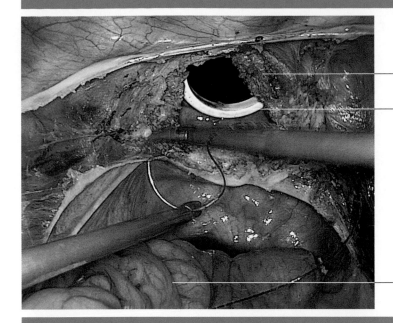

Resection margin

Ceramic ring of the manipulator

Colon

Closed vaginal cuff

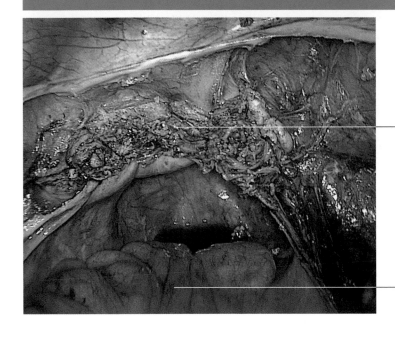

Vaginal cuff

Colon

11 Finishing the operation

T1 Laparoscope
T2 Atraumatic grasping forceps
T3 Suction and irrigation instrument
     Bipolar electrosurgical device
     Berci needle or 5/8 circle
     needle with small S-retractors

Sutures:
– Subcutaneous: 3–0 absorbable,
  multifilament or monofilament,
  as needed
– Skin: 3–0 absorbable,
  monofilament
– Skin adhesive

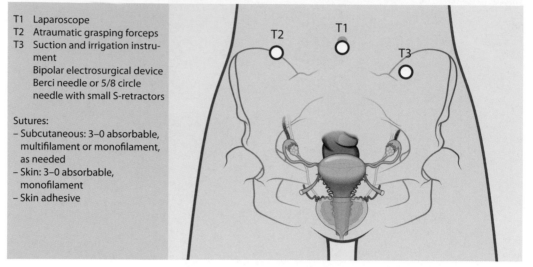

Using copious lavage to remove debris and clots, inspect the entire operating field carefully including all vascular pedicles, peritoneal edges, and the vesicovaginal plane. Use simple pressure or episodically delivered bipolar electrosurgery for hemostasis.

Ensure that the urine is not blood stained and the catheter not insufflated with CO_2.

Remove the accessory trocars (T2 and T3) carefully under direct vision. Bleeders can be controlled with pressure and time or a full thickness suture (→ **p. 57, V-1; V-2**).

> **Use copious lavage and inspect the entire operating field carefully. Inspect the urine in the catheter. Remove the accessory trocars under vision.**

> **Alternative: Placing a drain after difficult surgeries can be useful, however, there is evidence against placing routine drains, due to increased patients pain, prolonged hospital stay and adhesion formation.**

For a 12 mm accessory trocar, close the defect in a full thickness suture fashion under vision with a dedicated fascial closure device that closes both the fascial and peritoneal defects. A Berci needle provides the possibility to adapt the abdominal fascia under endoscopic view.

Remove the laparoscope (T1) and open the valve on the trocar for deflation. Then remove the trocar for the laparoscope. Close the fascia. Otherwise the defect can be sufficiently closed with a 5/8 circle needle (e.g. UR-6 needle) while exposed with small S retractors.

Close all cutaneous incisions by subcuticular absorbable monofilament suture (e.g. Monocryl®) and cover the wounds with sterile dressings.

> **Alternative: Instead of skin sutures and dressings, skin adhesive (e.g. Dermabond®) can be used to close the skin incisions.**

Consider performing cystoscopy at the end of the surgery with methylene blue dye given intravesically to evaluate the integrity of the ureters. Keep in mind that thermal injuries or necrosis may not appear on this test.

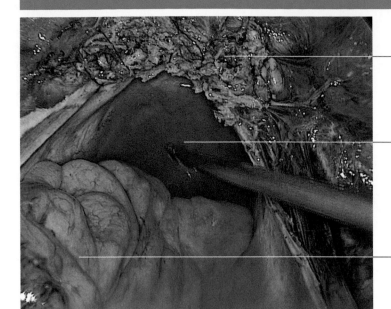

Vaginal cuff

Pouch of Douglas

Rectosigmoid Colon

Closing an incision

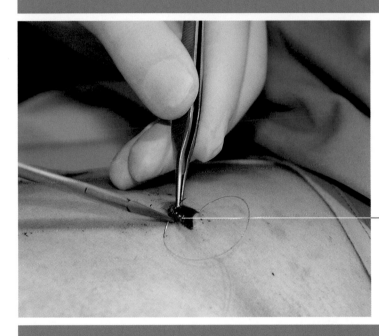

Skin incision for accessory trocar (5 mm)

Closing the umbilical incision

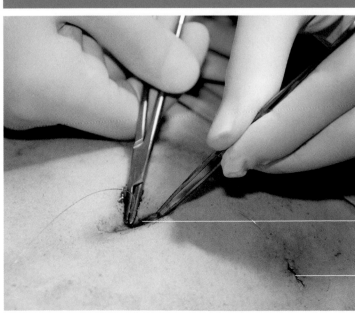

Umbilical incision

Closed skin incision

V   MANAGEMENT OF DIFFICULT SITUATIONS AND COMPLICATIONS

The threshold for converting to laparotomy, if necessary, should be adapted to the surgeon's experience in handling difficult situations. Convert immediately if the situation cannot be controlled laparoscopically!

1   Adhesions

Dissect adhesions by using an atraumatic forceps, scissors or ENSEAL® for tissue dissection. Work as close to the abdominal wall as possible to avoid organ injury. Respect dissection planes and minimize bleeding to prevent adhesion formation. Remove blood clots.

2   Blood vessel injuries

a) Diffuse bleeding/bleeding from minor vessels

Identify bleeding vessels and seal them with ENSEAL® or a regular bipolar device. If this does not terminate the bleeding, place a clip on the bleeding vessel.

b) Bleeding from major vessels

If larger vessels such as the iliac vessels, the aorta or vena cava are injured during the operation, use a blunt vascular clamp on the injury to reduce the bleeding. Proceed laparoscopically, depending on individual expertise. If in doubt, convert immediately to laparotomy and compress the vessel and treat the bleeding. Activate hospital protocol on major hemorrhage and consult for vascular surgical treatment, immediately.

3   Organ injuries

In case of injuries in which the extent cannot be determined with certainty, proceed to laparotomy. Open the abdominal cavity for assessment and management of the injury!

a) Greater omentum

Injury to the greater omentum can occur when the Veres needle is inserted too deeply and/or without elevation of the abdominal wall. Safety tests may not reveal a complication which can be identified with certainty only when the trocar and laparoscope are inserted.

Manage any bleeding that occurs with ENSEAL® or a regular bipolar device.

If, as a result of the insertion, the greater omentum is inflated like a tent, withdraw the trocar for the laparoscope to the peritoneal margin and tap the abdomen with an open hand. The omentum should then separate from the inside of the abdominal wall and collapse.

b) Bowel

Bowel injuries are usually caused by the first trocar or Veres needle that is inserted into the abdomen blindly. Beware of bowel injuries due to adhesions in case of previous surgeries and dense adhesions.

Manage bowel injuries by laparoscopic closure and oversewing with 3–0 absorbable polyfilament suture (e.g. Vicryl®). If sufficient closure of the injury is not guaranteed, perform a laparotomy. If necessary, convert to laparotomy and consult an urologist as per hospital protocol.

c) Ureter

Ureters should always be visualized and ureterolysis should be performed in difficult cases where the ureters may have an altered anatomical location. Keep in mind, that ureteric peristalsis is not a sign of integrity. In case of doubt, introduce a transurethral Double-J catheter. If necessary, convert to laparotomy and consult a urologist as per hospital protocol.

d) Urinary bladder

Detect injuries of the bladder by instilling diluted blue dye through the transurethral catheter. Manage injuries laparoscopically as in open surgery. A two-layer adaptation is recommended using 2–0 absorbable polyfilament suture (e.g. Vicryl®). If necessary, convert to laparotomy and consult a urologist as per hospital protocol.

4   Preperitoneal air emphysema

a) Veres needle

An insufficient CO_2 gas flow may result from an incorrectly placed needle. Remove the needle and reinsert it as described above (→ **p. 27, IIa**). Ensure particularly that the angle of insertion is vertical and that the abdominal wall is lifted. Use the Palmer's Point entry (left upper quadrant laparoscopic entry), if no adequate pneumoperitoneum can be established.

b) Trocar

If the tip of the insufflating trocar is placed subcutaneously, push the tip of the trocar through the peritoneum in the abdominal cavity.

5   Losing a swab in the abdominal cavity

After losing a swab, fix the trocar in its last position and locate the swab with direct visualization. Use an atraumatic grasping forceps.

Do not change the patient's position, and do not irrigate the abdominal cavity!

If necessary, search for the swab with the C-arm or perform a laparotomy to retrieve the swab.

APPENDICES

Anatomical variations

a) Uterine artery
b) Uterus

Variation of the laparoscopic hysterectomy: Laparoscopic supracervical hysterectomy (LSH)

7. Resecting the uterine fundus
8. Removing the uterine corpus

Sample operation notes

a) Total laparoscopic hysterectomy
b) Laparoscopic supracervical hysterectomy

Potential operating steps

a) Salpingo-oophorectomy
b) Opening the retroperitoneum and exposing the uterine artery crossing the ureter

Postoperative management

a) Analgesia
b) Mobilization
c) Nutrition
d) Diagnostics
e) Discharge
f) Recommendations to the patient

Management of postoperative complications

a) Postoperative bleeding
b) Infection
c) Vaginal cuff dehiscence

APPENDICES

- Bibliography

- Alphabetical index

- Editors

- Assistants

- Titles available

a) Uterine artery

The uterine artery branches into descending and ascending vessels, communicating with vaginal and ovarian vessels. Their course is meandering so that they can stretch with uterine enlargement during pregnancy. Be aware of this while manipulating.

b) Uterus

If the uterus is massively enlarged or a patient is notably small and obese, consider placing the trocar for the laparoscope at the Lee-Huang point (midline, 3–4 cm above the umbilicus), in order to allow adequate visibility and manipulation of instruments.

Variation of laparoscopic hysterectomy: Laparoscopic supracervical hysterectomy (LSH)

01 Exploring the abdominal cavity

02 Identifying the anatomical landmarks

03 Transecting the round ligament

04 Transecting the ovarian ligament and the Fallopian tube

05 Dissecting the broad ligament

06 Identifying the ureter

07 Resecting the uterine fundus

08 Removing the uterine corpus

11 Finishing the operation

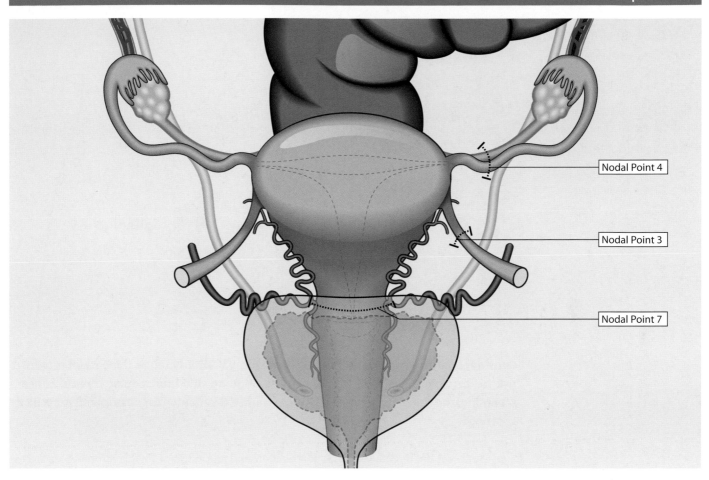

Nodal Point 4

Nodal Point 3

Nodal Point 7

Variation of laparoscopic hysterectomy: LSH

Perform nodal points 1 to 6 as described on pages 34–45.

7 Resecting the uterine fundus

T1   Laparoscope
T2   Monopolar hook or ENSEAL®
     G2 Curved & Straight Tissue
     Sealers (or T3)
T3   Atraumatic grasping forceps
     (or T2)

– Ring forceps
– Suture: 2–0
  absorbable, monofilament or
  multifilament, as needed

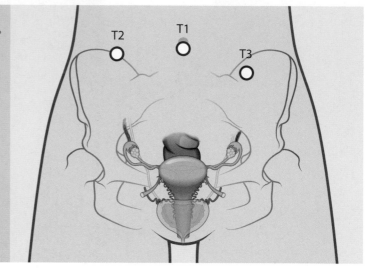

Consider laparoscopic supracervical hysterectomy (LSH) as long as the patient is at low risk for cervical cancer and is aware of the ongoing need for regular cervical cancer screening, the risk of future cervical descent, and the potential for postoperative cyclical spotting.

Expose and seal the uterine vessels as described in nodal point 7 for total laparoscopic hysterectomy, except for extending the peritoneal dissection around the posterior aspect of the cervix.

Once the fundus has turned a dusky blue, both uterine vessels have been sufficiently prepared for excision of the fundus from the underlying cervix.

Avoid inadvertent entry into the vagina or uterosacral complex by incising just above the nexus of the uterosacral ligament with the pericervical ring at the level of the true uterine isthmus.

Avoid inadvertent entry into the vagina or uterosacral complex.

Resect the fundus using monopolar electrosurgery or ENSEAL®.

Shape the stump intentionally into a reverse cone shape during resection, to minimize the chance of residual endometrial tissue.

Remove the uterine manipulator before completing the resection. Place a ring forceps with a folded gauze sponge to elevate and manipulate the cervical stump thereafter.

Control small bleeders by the episodic application of bipolar electrosurgery using the tips to touch and tamponade before desiccating. Moreover, desiccate the endocervix circumferentially with bipolar electrosurgery to minimize the chance of postoperative cyclical spotting.

To reduce the chance of postoperative adhesion formation to the cervical stump, the peritoneal defect may be closed with a running suture using absorbable monofilament or multifilament suture. There is no need to suture the stromal defect in the cervical stump.

Urinary bladder

Uterine cervix

Fundus

Rectosigmoid colon

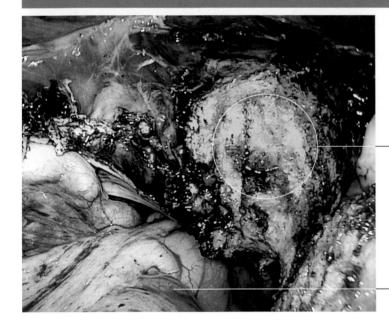

Cervical stump

Rectosigmoid colon

8 Removing the uterine corpus

T1   Laparoscope
T2   Monopolar hook (or T3)
T3   Atraumatic grasping forceps (or T2)

– Atraumatic grasping forceps
– Swab as needed
– Needle holder as needed
– Size 11 scalpel as needed

Sutures:
– Vagina: 2 – 0 absorbable mono-filament as needed
– Subcutaneous: 3 – 0 absorbable, multifilament or monofilament, as needed
– Skin: 3 – 0 absorbable, mono-filament as needed

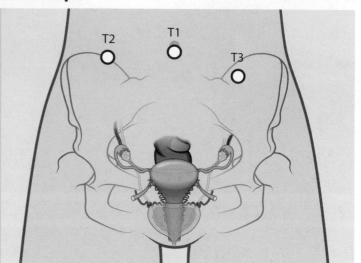

After resecting the corpus, evaluate whether the corpus size can be removed through a culdotomy or whether a Pfannenstiel incision of the abdominal wall is required.

For a transvaginal removal, insert a swab through the vagina into the posterior fornix as a counter bearing. Laparoscopically incise the posterior fornix transversally. Remove the swab followed by the uterine corpus through the vagina. Continuously suture the incision either laparoscopically or transvaginally with 2–0 absorbable monofilament.

In case of a larger uterine corpus, perform a standard Pfannenstiel transverse incision according to your hospital protocol.

Alternative: Exchange the left accessory trocar for a morcellator. Morcellate the uterine corpus under vision. Make sure that all uterine tissue is extracted from the abdominal cavity.

The FDA (USA) warns that uterine tissue may contain unsuspected cancer. The use of laparoscopic power morcellators during fibroid surgery may spread cancer, and decrease the long-term survival of patients. Share this information with patients when considering morcellation.

To finish the operation, perform nodal point 11 (→ **p. 54, IV**).

Incising the abdominal wall above the pubic symphysis (Pfannenstiel incision)

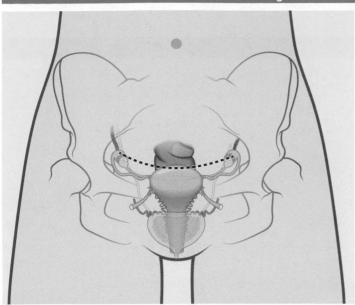

Suturing the incision of the posterior vaginal fornix

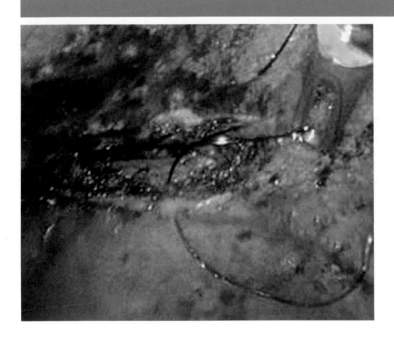

Sample operation notes

a) Total laparoscopic hysterectomy (TLH)

Date:	Operating surgeon:
Patient's name:	Assistant:
Operation diagnosis:	Scrub nurse:
Operation:	Anesthetist:

Identification of patient, disinfection, sterile drapes and indwelling urinary catheter.

Insertion of uterine manipulator into uterine corpus.

Vertical incision at base of umbilicus and insertion of Veres needle. Semm safety tests. CO_2 insufflation to intra-abdominal pressure of 20 mmHg. Removal of Veres needle and insertion of trocar for the laparoscope. Lithotomy position.

Inspection of abdomen. Upper abdominal organs without abnormalities.

Insertion of 2 x 5mm accessory trocars under vision lateral to superficial epigastric vessels in left and right lower abdomen.

Normal sized uterus with normal ovaries and tubes. Peritoneum without abnormalities. Adhesions in right lower abdomen after appendectomy.

Identification and coagulation of round ligament. Coagulation of ovarian ligament and tube.

Opening of broad ligament and retroperitoneum to identify the ureter. Ureterolysis. Further dissection of broad ligament and opening of bladder peritoneum and dissection of bladder downwards.

Same procedure on the contralateral side. Skeletonizing of cervix.

Insertion of uterine manipulator cuff and transection of uterus and transvaginal removal.

Closure of vaginal vault with intracorporeal suturing of vagina using absorbable monofilament running suture (e.g. PDS® 0, Ethicon Products).

Hemostasis ensured after irrigation and suction of fluids.

Retraction of trocars under vision, deflation of pneumoperitoneum. Closure of 10 mm trocar for the laparoscope site fascia with absorbable polyfilament (e.g. Vicryl® 2–0).

Intracutaneous suture with absorbable monofilament (e.g. Monocryl® 3–0, Ethicon Products) and skin adhesive (e.g. Dermabond®) dressing.

The urine is clear, estimated blood loss 50 ml.

b) Laparoscopic supracervical hysterectomy (LSH)

Date:	Operating surgeon:
Patient's name:	Assistant:
Operation diagnosis:	Scrub nurse:
Operation:	Anesthetist:

Identification of patient, disinfection, sterile drapes and indwelling urinary catheter.

Insertion of uterine manipulator into uterine corpus.

Vertical incision at base of umbilicus and insertion of Veres needle. Semm safety tests. CO_2 insufflation to intra-abdominal pressure of 20 mmHg. Removal of Veres needle and insertion of optical trocar. Lithotomy position.

Inspection of abdomen. Upper abdominal organs without abnormalities.

Insertion of 2 x 5 mm accessory trocars under vision lateral to superficial epigastric vessels in left and right lower abdomen.

Normal sized uterus with normal ovaries and tubes. Peritoneum without abnormalities. Adhesions in right lower abdomen after appendectomy.

Identification and coagulation of left round ligament. Coagulation of ovarian ligament and tube.

Opening of broad ligament and retroperitoneum to identify the ureter. Further dissection of broad ligament and coagulation of uterine arteries.

Same procedure on the contralateral side and defining plane to transect the uterine fundus.

Removal of uterine manipulator and transection of uterine fundus.

Thorough coagulation of cervical canal with bipolar forceps.

Transverse incision in the posterior fornix, transvaginal removal of the uterine corpus.

Laparoscopic closure with absorbable monofilament suture.

Hemostasis ensured after irrigation and suction of fluids.

Retraction of trocars under vision, deflation of pneumoperitoneum. Closure of 10 mm trocar site with absorbable polyfilament (e.g. Vicryl® 2–0).

Intracutaneous suture with absorbable monofilament (e.g. Monocryl® 3–0, Ethicon Products) and skin adhesive (e.g. Dermabond®) dressing.

The urine is clear, estimated blood loss 50 ml.

a) Salpingo-oophorectomy

Discuss with the individual patient whether ovaries without pathology should be removed. If indicated, after transecting the round ligament (→ **p. 38, IV-3**) and visualizing the ureter, seal the infundibulopelvic ligament proximally and distally before transecting because of concomitant blood vessels. A slight blanching of the tissue should be visible. Transect the infundibulopelvic ligament between the sealed streaks by slowly advancing the ENSEAL® I-BLADE® until it reaches the distal end of the jaw.

Round ligament

Fallopian tube

Ligamentum infundibulopelvicum, proximal stump

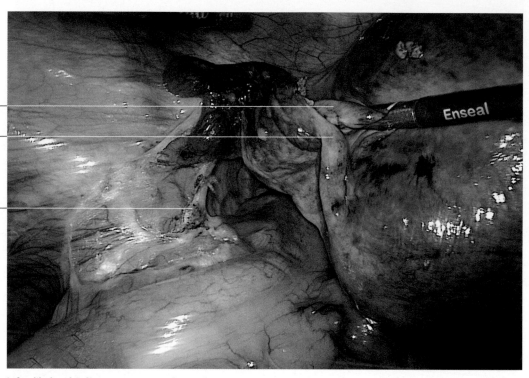

Infundibulopelvic ligament transected

b) Opening the retroperitoneum and exposing the uterine artery crossing the ureter

For better comprehension of the anatomical situation, especially in obese women and with enlarged uteri, it may be helpful to open the retroperitoneum and expose the uterine artery and the ureter.

Open the retroperitoneum after transecting the round ligament (→ **p. 38, IV-3**) and before transecting the ovarian ligament and the Fallopian tube (→ **p. 40, IV-4**).

Identify the ureter, and expose the uterine artery as it crosses the ureter.

Identify and pull the umbilical ligament to simplify detection of the internal iliac artery and thereby the first medial branch (the uterine artery).

Seal the uterine vessels to reduce bleeding during the following steps. Continue dissecting the broad ligament (→ **p. 42, IV-5**).

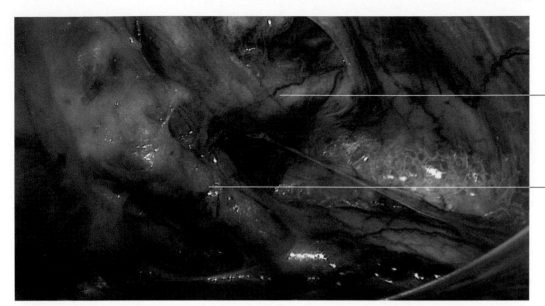

Ureter

Uterine vessels

Uterine vessels crossing the ureter

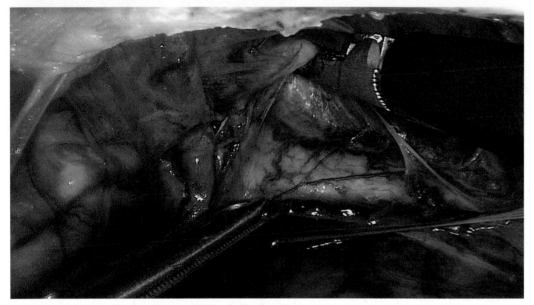

Uterine artery (held by ENSEAL® instrument) and ureter below

Postoperative management

a) Analgesia

Take care to give adequate pain medication for faster recovery of the patient.

Rely on standardized postoperative analgesia protocols of your hospital and ask your patient to report inadequate pain control.

b) Mobilization

Mobilize the patient as soon as possible in order to reduce postoperative complications, ideally on the evening following surgery.

c) Nutrition

Let the patient drink and eat on the evening following surgery. Rely on fast-track surgery recommendations and your hospital protocol.

d) Diagnostics

Intensive care observation is rarely necessary after TLH or LSH but may be necessary due to the patient's individual risk factors and comorbidities.

> **Conduct the usual postoperative monitoring and care, including blood count on the day of surgery.**

e) Discharge

Discharge the patient between the second and fifth postoperative day. Make sure that the patient is mobile, is urinating freely, has adequate pain control, and does not have excessive vaginal bleeding.

> **Prior to discharge conduct transvaginal sonography and sonography of the kidneys to rule out hydronephrosis.**

f) Recommendations to the patient

Inform the patient that she should not lift heavy burdens for at least two weeks and should allow for vaginal wound healing prior to sexual intercourse – not earlier than four to six weeks after surgery.

Management of postoperative complications

a) Postoperative bleeding

If postoperative intra-abdominal bleeding is suspected, perform a laparoscopy in order to locate and stop the bleeding.

If there is bleeding from the vaginal cuff, consider transvaginal overstitching.

b) Infection

Surgical wound infections are the most common postoperative complications. Start treatment according to hospital protocol (metronidazole or cephalosporin).

Perfom transvaginal sonography to rule out an abscess inside the pelvis. Decide if surgical re-evaluation is necessary.

c) Vaginal cuff dehiscence

Vaginal cuff dehiscence is a rare postoperative complication.

Reduce risk for vaginal cuff dehiscence by transvaginal inspection of every laparoscopically sutured vaginal cuff during the learning phase. If necessary, perform a vaginal adaptation subsequently.

In case of secondary vaginal cuff dehiscence, rule out an infection before attempting another surgical closure.

Bibliography

Al-Talib A., Sheizaf B., Almog B., Dawood A., Krishnamurthy S. & Tulandi T. (2011). Morbidity with total laparoscopic and laparoscopically assisted vaginal hysterectomy. *Acta Obstetricia et Gynecologica Scandinavica,* 90: 284–287.

Arora S., Aggarwal R., Sevdalis N., Moran A., Sirimanna P., Kneebone R. & Darzi A. (2010). Development and validation of mental practice as a training strategy for laparoscopic surgery. *Surgical Endoscopy,* 24: 179–187.

Bijen C.B., de Bock G.H., Vermeulen K.M., Arts H.J., Ter Brugge H.G., van der Sijde R., Kraayenbrink A.A., Bongers M.Y., van der Zee A.G. & Mourits M.J. (2011). Laparoscopic hysterectomy is preferred over laparotomy in early endometrial cancer patients, however not cost effective in the very obese. *European Journal of Cancer,* 47: 2158-2165.

Bijen C.B., Vermeulen K.M., Mourits M.J. & de Bock G.H. (2009). Costs and effects of abdominal versus laparoscopic hysterectomy: systematic review of controlled trials. *Public Library of Science One,* 4: e7340.

Bojahr B., Tchartchian G. & Ohlinger R. (2009). Laparoscopic supracervical hysterectomy: a retrospective analysis of 1000 cases. *Journal of the Society of Laparoendoscopic Surgeons,* 13: 129–134.

Boyd L.R., Novetsky A.P. & Curtin J.P. (2010). Effect of surgical volume on route of hysterectomy and short-term morbidity. *Obstetrics & Gynecology,* 116: 909–915.

Candiani M. & Izzo S. (2010). Laparoscopic versus vaginal hysterectomy for benign pathology. *Current Opinion in Obstetrics and Gynecology,* 22: 304–308.

Carpenter W.B. (1874). *Principles of Mental Physiology: With their Applications to the Training and Discipline of the Mind and the Study of its Comorbid Conditions.* London: Henry S. King & Co.

Chesson R.R. (2011). Cystoscopy should be a routine procedure in the performance of hysterectomy. *Journal of Reproductive Medicine,* 56: 373–375.

Cipullo L., De Paoli S., Fasolino L. & Fasolino A. (2009). Laparoscopic supracervical hysterectomy compared to total hysterectomy. *Journal of the Society of Laparoendoscopic Surgeons,* 13: 370–375.

de Lapasse C., Rabischong B., Bolandard F., Canis M., Botchorischvili R., Jardon K. & Mage G. (2008). Total laparoscopic hysterectomy and early discharge: satisfaction and feasibility study. *Journal of Minimally Invasive Gynecology,* 15: 20–25.

Donnez O., Jadoul P., Squifflet J. & Donnez J. (2009). A series of 3190 laparoscopic hysterectomies for benign disease from 1990 to 2006: evaluation of complications compared with vaginal and abdominal procedures. *British Journal of Obstetrics and Gynaecology,* 116: 492–500.

Drahonovsky J., Haakova L., Otcenasek M., Krofta L., Kucera E. & Feyereisl J. (2010). A prospective randomized comparison of vaginal hysterectomy, laparoscopically assisted vaginal hysterectomy, and total laparoscopic hysterectomy in women with benign uterine disease. *European Journal of Obstetrics & Gynecology and Reproductive Biology,* 148: 172–176.

Einarsson J.I. & Suzuki Y. (2009). Total laparoscopic hysterectomy: 10 steps toward a successful procedure. *Reviews in Obstetrics and Gynecology*, 2: 57–64.

Feltz D.L. & Landers D.M. (1983). The effects of mental practice on motor skill learning and performance: a meta-analysis. *Journal of Sport Psychology*, 5: 25–57.

Frumovitz M. (2010). Laparoscopic total hysterectomy vs supracervical hysterectomy: turn, turn, turn. *Journal of Minimally Invasive Gynecology*, 17: 669–670.

Gendy R., Walsh C.A., Walsh S.R. & Karantanis E. (2011). Vaginal hysterectomy versus total laparoscopic hysterectomy for benign disease: a metaanalysis of randomized controlled trials. *American Journal of Obstetrics & Gynecology*, 204: 388.e1–8.

Ghezzi F,. Uccella S., Cromi A., Siesto G., Serati M., Bogani G. & Bolis P. (2010). Postoperative pain after laparoscopic and vaginal hysterectomy for benign gynecologic disease: a randomized trial. *American Journal of Obstetrics & Gynecology*, 203: 118.e1–8.

Güler A.K., Immenroth M., Berg T., Bürger T. & Gawad K.A. (2006). Evaluation einer neu konzipierten Operationsfibel durch den Vergleich mit einer klassischen chirurgischen Operationslehre. *Posterpräsentation auf dem 123. Kongress der Deutschen Gesellschaft für Chirurgie* vom 02.–05. Mai 2006 in Berlin.

Hamilton B., McClellan S.N., Rettenmaier M.A. & Goldstein B.H. (2009). Laparoscopic supracervical hysterectomy for benign gynecologic conditions. *Journal of the Society of Laparoendoscopic Surgeons*, 13: 19–21.

Harmanli O.H., Tunitsky E., Esin S., Citil A. & Knee A. (2009). A comparison of short-term outcomes between laparoscopic supracervical and total hysterectomy. *American Journal of Obstetrics & Gynecology*, 201: 536.e1–7.

Heaton R.L. & Walid M.S. (2010). An intention-to-treat study of total laparoscopic hysterectomy. *International Journal of Gynecology & Obstetrics*, 111: 57–61.

Hohl M.K. & Hauser N. (2010). Safe total intrafascial laparoscopic (TAIL) hysterectomy: a prospective cohort study. *Gynecological Surgery*, 7: 231–239.

Hwang J.H., Lee J.K., Lee N.W. & Lee K.W. (2011). Vaginal cuff closure: a comparison between the vaginal route and laparoscopic suture in patients undergoing total laparoscopic hysterectomy. *Gynecologic and Obstetric Investigation*, 71: 163–169.

Immenroth M. (2003). *Mentales Training in der Medizin. Anwendung in der Chirurgie und Zahnmedizin.* Hamburg: Kovac.

Immenroth M., Bürger T., Brenner J., Kemmler R., Nagelschmidt R., Eberspächer H. & Troidl H. (2005). Mentales Training in der Chirurgie. *Der Chirurg BDC*, 44: 21–25.

Immenroth M., Bürger T., Brenner J., Nagelschmidt R., Eberspächer H. & Troidl H. (2007). Mental Training in surgical education: a randomized controlled trial. *Annals of Surgery*, 245: 385–391.

Immenroth M., Eberspächer H. & Hermann H.D. (2008). Training kognitiver Fertigkeiten. In J. Beckmann & M. Kellmann (Hrsg.), *Enzyklopädie der Psychologie (D, V, 2). Anwendungen der Sportpsychologie* (119–176). Göttingen: Hogrefe.

Immenroth M., Eberspächer H., Nagelschmidt M., Troidl H., Bürger T., Brenner J., Berg T., Müller M. & Kemmler R. (2005). Mentales Training in der Chirurgie – Sicherheit durch ein besseres Training. Design und erste Ergebnisse einer Studie. *MIC,* 14: 69–74.

Janda M., Gebski V., Brand A., Hogg R., Jobling T.W,. Land R., Manolitsas T., McCartney A., Nascimento M., Neesham D., Nicklin J.L., Oehler M.K., Otton G., Perrin L., Salfinger S., Hammond I., Leung Y., Walsh T., Sykes P., Ngan H., Garrett A., Laney M., Ng T.Y., Tam K., Chan K., Wrede C.D., Pather S., Simcock B., Farrell R. & Obermair A. (2010). Quality of life after total laparoscopic hysterectomy versus total abdominal hysterectomy for stage I endometrial cancer (LACE): a randomised trial. *Lancet Oncology,* 11: 772–780.

Jelovsek J.E., Chiung C., Chen G., Roberts S.L., Paraiso M.F. & Falcone T. (2007). Incidence of lower urinary tract injury at the time of total laparoscopic hysterectomy. *Journal of the Society of Laparoendoscopic Surgeons,* 11: 422–427.

Johnson N., Barlow D., Lethaby A., Tavender E., Curr E. & Garry R. (2006). Surgical approach to hysterectomy for benign gynaecological disease. *Cochrane Database of Systematic Reviews,* 19: CD003677.

Jonsdottir G.M., Jorgensen S., Cohen S.L., Wright K.N., Shah N.T., Chavan N. & Einarsson J.I. (2011). Increasing minimally invasive hysterectomy: effect on cost and complications. *Obstetrics & Gynecology,* 117: 1142–1149.

Kafy S., Al-Sannan B., Kabli N. & Tulandi T. (2009). Patient satisfaction after laparoscopic total or supracervical hysterectomy. *Gynecologic and Obstetric Investigation,* 67: 169–172.

Kives S., Lefebvre G., Wolfman W., Leyland N., Allaire C., Awadalla A., Best C., Leroux N., Potestio F., Rittenberg D., Soucy R. & Singh S. (2010). Supracervical hysterectomy. *Journal of Obstetrics and Gynaecology Canada,* 32: 62–68.

Krizova A., Clarke B.A., Bernardini M.Q., James S., Kalloger S.E., Boerner S.L. & Mulligan A.M. (2011). Histologic artifacts in abdominal, vaginal, laparoscopic, and robotic hysterectomy specimens: a blinded, retrospective review. *American Journal of Surgical Pathology,* 35: 115–126.

Laberge P.Y. & Singh S.S. (2009). Surgical approach to hysterectomy: introducing the concept of technicity. *Journal of Obstetrics and Gynaecology Canada,* 31: 1050–1053.

Lafay Pillet M.C., Leonard F., Chopin N., Malaret J.M., Borghese B., Foulot H., Fotso A. & Chapron C. (2009). Incidence and risk factors of bladder injuries during laparoscopic hysterectomy indicated for benign uterine pathologies: a 14.5 years experience in a continuous series of 1501 procedures. *Human Reproduction,* 24: 842–849.

Lotze R.H. (1852). *Medicinische Psychologie und Physiologie der Seele.* Leipzig: Weidmann'sche Buchhandlung.

McCartney A.J. & Obermair A. (2004). Total laparoscopic hysterectomy with a transvaginal tube. *The Journal of the American Association of Gynecologic Laparoscopists*, 11: 79–82.

McPherson K., Metcalfe M.A., Herbert A., Maresh M., Casbard A., Hargreaves J., Bridgman S. & Clarke A. (2004). Severe complications of hysterectomy: the VALUE study. *British Journal of Obstetrics and Gynaecology*, 111: 688–694.

Miller G.A. (1956). The magical number seven plus or minus two: some limits on our capacity for processing information. *Psychological Review*, 63: 81–97.

Minelli L., Franciolini G., Franchini M.A., Mutolo F. & Momoli G. (1990) [Laparoscopic hysterectomy]. *Minerva Ginecologica*, 42: 515–518.

Mousa A., Zarei A. & Tulandi T. (2009). Changing practice from laparoscopic supracervical hysterectomy to total hysterectomy. *Journal of Obstetrics and Gynaecology Canada*, 31: 521–525.

Mueller A., Boosz A,. Koch M., Jud S., Faschingbauer F., Schrauder M., Löhberg C., Mehlhorn G., Renner S.P,. Lux M.P., Beckmann M.W. & Thiel F.C. (2011). The Hohl instrument for optimizing total laparoscopic hysterectomy: results of more than 500 procedures in a university training center. *Archives of Gynecology and Obstetrics*, 285: 123–127.

Mueller A., Renner S.P., Haeberle L., Lermann J., Oppelt P., Beckmann M.W. & Thiel F. (2009). Comparison of total laparoscopic hysterectomy (TLH) and laparoscopy-assisted supracervical hysterectomy (LASH) in women with uterine leiomyoma. *European Journal of Obstetrics & Gynecology and Reproductive Biology*, 144: 76–79.

Mueller A., Thiel F.C., Renner S.P., Winkler M., Haeberle L. & Beckmann M.W. (2010). Hysterectomy – A comparison of approaches. *Deutsches Ärzteblatt international*, 107: 353–359.

Nascimento M.C., Kelley A., Martitsch C., Weidner I. & Obermair A. (2005). Postoperative analgesic requirements – total laparoscopic hysterectomy versus vaginal hysterectomy. *The Australian and New Zealand Journal of Obstetrics and Gynaecology*, 45: 140–143.

Nawfal A.K., Orady M., Eisenstein D. & Wegienka G. (2011). Effect of body mass index on robotic-assisted total laparoscopic hysterectomy. *Journal of Minimally Invasive Gynecology*, 18: 328–332.

Obermair A., Janda M., Baker J., Kondalsamy-Chennakesavan S., Brand A., Hogg R., Jobling T.W., Land R., Manolitsas T., Nascimento M., Neesham D., Nicklin J.L., Oehler M.K., Otton G., Perrin L., Salfinger S., Hammond I., Leung Y., Sykes P., Ngan H., Garrett A., Laney M., Ng T.Y., Tam K., Chan K., Wrede D.H., Pather S., Simcock B., Farrell R., Robertson G., Walker G., McCartney A. & Gebski V. (2012). Improved surgical safety after laparoscopic compared to open surgery for apparent early stage endometrial cancer: Results from a randomised controlled trial. *European Journal of Cancer*, 48: 1147–1153.

O'Hanlan K.A., Dibble S.L., Garnier A.C. & Reuland M.L. (2007). Total laparoscopic hysterectomy: technique and complications of 830 cases. *Journal of the Society of Laparoendoscopic Surgeons*, 11: 45–53.

O'Hanlan K.A., McCutcheon S.P. & McCutcheon J.G. (2011). Laparoscopic hysterectomy: impact of uterine size. *Journal of Minimally Invasive Gynecology*, 18: 85–91.

Park S.H., Cho H.Y. & Kim H.B. (2011). Factors determining conversion to laparotomy in patients undergoing total laparoscopic hysterectomy. *Gynecologic and Obstetric Investigation,* 71: 193–197.

Parker W.H. (2004). Total laparoscopic hysterectomy and laparoscopic supracervical hysterectomy. *Obstetrics & Gynecology Clinics of North America,* 31: 523–537, viii.

Reich H. (2007). Total laparoscopic hysterectomy: indications, techniques and outcomes. *Current Opinion in Obstetrics and Gynecology,* 19: 337–344.

Reich H. (1992). Laparoscopic hysterectomy. *Surgical Laparoscopy, Endoscopy & Percutaneous Techniques,* 2: 85–88.

Roman H., Zanati J., Friederich L., Resch B., Lena E. & Marpeau L. (2008). Laparoscopic hysterectomy of large uteri with uterine artery coagulation at its origin. *Journal of the Society of Laparoendoscopic Surgeons,* 12: 25–29.

Schmidt T., Eren Y., Breidenbach M., Fehr D., Volkmer A., Fleisch M. & Rein D.T. (2011). Modifications of laparoscopic supracervical hysterectomy technique significantly reduce postoperative spotting. *Journal of Minimally Invasive Gynecology,* 18: 81–84.

Sinha R., Sundaram M., Lakhotia S., Hedge A. & Kadam P. (2010). Total laparoscopic hysterectomy in women with previous cesarean sections. *Journal of Minimally Invasive Gynecology,* 17: 513–517.

Sinha R., Sundaram M., Mahajan C., Raje S., Kadam P., Rao G. & Shitut P. (2011). Single-incision total laparoscopic hysterectomy. *Journal of Minimal Access Surgery,* 7: 78–82.

Song J.Y., Hwang S.J., Kim M.J., Jo H.H., Kim S.Y., Choi K.E., Kwon D.J., Lew Y.O., Kim J.H., Lim Y.T., Kim J.H., Kim E.J. & Kim M.R. (2010). Comparison of selective uterine artery double ligation at the isthmic level of uterus and bipolar uterine artery coagulation in total laparoscopic hysterectomy. *Minimally Invasive Therapy & Allied Technologies,* 19: 224–230.

Song T., Kim T.J., Kang H., Lee Y.Y., Choi C.H., Lee J.W., Kim B.G. & Bae D.S. (2011). A review of the technique and complications from 2,012 cases of laparoscopically assisted vaginal hysterectomy at a single institution. *The Australian and New Zealand Journal of Obstetrics and Gynaecology,* 51: 239–243.

Sutton C. (2010). Past, present, and future of hysterectomy. *Journal of Minimally Invasive Gynecology,* 17: 421–435.

Thangaswamy C.R., Rewari V,. Trikha A,. Dehran M. & Chandralekha. (2010). Dexamethasone before total laparoscopic hysterectomy: a randomized controlled dose-response study. *Journal of Anesthesia,* 24: 24–30.

Tchartchian G., Dietzel J., Bojahr B., Hackethal A. & De Wilde R.L. (2010). No more abdominal hysterectomy for myomata using a new minimally-invasive technique. *International Journal of Surgery Case Reports,* 1: 7–8.

Thiel J. & Gamelin A. (2003). Outpatient total laparoscopic hysterectomy. *The Journal of the American Association of Gynecologic Laparoscopists,* 10: 481–483.

U. S. Food and Drug Administration. (2014). Updated laparoscopic uterine power morcellation in hysterectomy and myomectomy: FDA safety communication. http://www.fda.gov/MedicalDevices/Safety/AlertsandNotices/ucm424443.htm

Van Evert J.S., Smeenk J.M., Dijkhuizen F.P., de Kruif J.H. & Kluivers K.B. (2010). Laparoscopic subtotal hysterectomy versus laparoscopic total hysterectomy: a decade of experience. *Gynecological Surgery*, 7: 9–12.

Walid M.S. & Heaton R.L. (2010). Promoting awareness about total laparoscopic hysterectomy. *Southern Medical Journal*, 103: 98.

Walid M.S. & Heaton R.L. (2010). Total laparoscopic hysterectomy for uteri over one kilogram. *Journal of the Society of Laparoendoscopic Surgeons*, 14: 178–182.

Walsh C.A., Walsh S.R., Tang T.Y. & Slack M. (2009). Total abdominal hysterectomy versus total laparoscopic hysterectomy for benign disease: a meta-analysis. *European Journal of Obstetrics & Gynecology and Reproductive Biology*, 144: 3–7.

Marc Immenroth, PhD

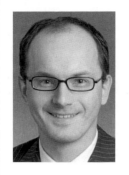

- Studied psychology (Diploma) and sports science (Master) in Heidelberg, Germany
- 1999–2006 Sports psychologist (including consultant to many German top athletes during their preparation for the World Championships and Olympics) and industrial psychologist (including consultant to Lufthansa Inc.)
- 2000 Research scientist at the University of Greifswald, Germany (Polyclinic for Restorative Dentistry and Periodontology)
- 2001–2004 Research scientist at the University of Heidelberg, Germany (Institute of Sports and Sports Science)
- 2002 Doctorate in psychology at the University of Heidelberg, Germany
- 2005–2006 Assistant lecturer at the University of Giessen, Germany (Institute of Sports)
- 2006–2008 Assistant professor at the University of Greifswald, Germany (Institute of Sports)
- 2006–2009 European Clinical Studies Manager at Ethicon Endo-Surgery (Europe) GmbH in Norderstedt, Germany
- 2009–2012 Marketing Manager and Sales Support at Ethicon Products, Johnson & Johnson Medical GmbH in Norderstedt, Germany
- 2012–2014 Marketing Manager Ethicon Surgical Care, Johnson & Johnson Medical GmbH in Norderstedt, Germany
- Since 2014 Sales & Business Development Manager Ethicon Surgical Care, Johnson & Johnson Medical GmbH in Norderstedt, Germany

Focus of Research and Work
- Mental training in sports, surgery and aviation
- Virtual reality in surgical education
- Coping with emotion and stress

Author of many scientific articles and textbooks on psychology, sports science and medicine.

Jürgen Brenner, MD

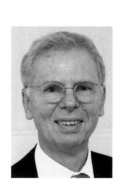

- Studied medicine in Hamburg, Germany
- 1972 Doctorate in medicine at the University of Hamburg, Germany
- 1972 Institute for Neuroanatomy, University of Hamburg, Germany
- 1974 Senior Resident at the Department of Surgery of the General Hospital Hamburg-Wandsbek, Germany
- 1981 Medical Director of the Department for Colorectal and Trauma Surgery at St. Adolf Stift Hospital in Reinbek, Germany
- 1987 Director for Surgical Research of Ethicon Inc. in Norderstedt, Germany
- 1989 Director of European Surgical Institute and Vice President Professional Education Europe of Ethicon Endo-Surgery (Europe) GmbH in Norderstedt, Germany
- 2004 Managing Director at Ethicon Endo-Surgery Germany in Norderstedt, Germany
- 2008–2011 Director of European Surgical Institute in Norderstedt, Germany
- Since 2011 Managing Director, Eric Krauthammer & Dr. Jürgen Brenner, Creative Team-Leadership

Assistants

Dr. Carl GmbH

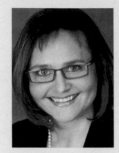

Ellen Markert, MD
Medical Writer

European Surgical Institute (ESI)

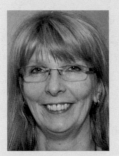

Maike Aukstinnis
Team Coordinator
Medical Training

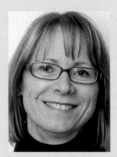

Annegret Röhling
Project Coordinator

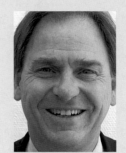

Detlev Ruge
Manager Event Technology

ETHICON Surgical Care Johnson & Johnson MEDICAL GmbH

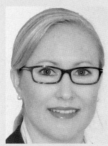

Ann-Katrin Bruns, née Güler, MD
Consultant Medical Products

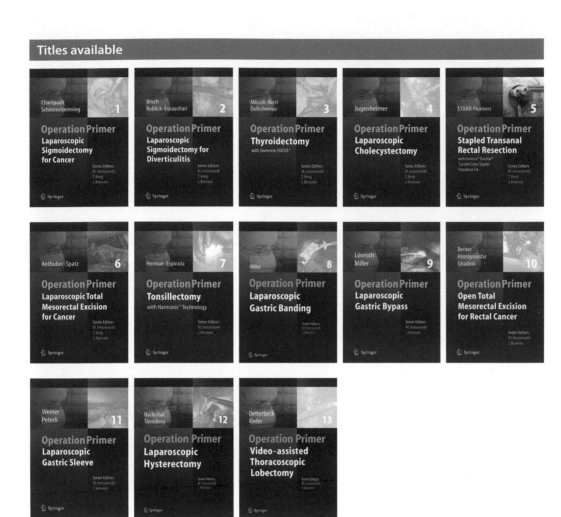

Volume 1:	Laparoscopic Sigmoidectomy for Cancer	ISBN 978-3-540-78453-1
Volume 2:	Laparoscopic Sigmoidectomy for Diverticulitis	ISBN 978-3-540-78451-7
Volume 3:	Thyroidectomy with Harmonic FOCUS®	ISBN 978-3-540-85163-9
Volume 4:	Laparoscopic Cholecystectomy	ISBN 978-3-540-92961-1
Volume 5:	Stapled Transanal Rectal Resection with Contour® Transtar™ Curved Cutter Stapler Procedure Set	ISBN 978-3-540-92958-1
Volume 6:	Laparoscopic Total Mesorectal Excision for Cancer	ISBN 978-3-642-04730-5
Volume 7:	Tonsillectomy with Harmonic® Technology	ISBN 978-3-642-12747-2
Volume 8:	Laparoscopic Gastric Banding	ISBN 978-3-642-19274-6
Volume 9:	Laparoscopic Gastric Bypass	ISBN 978-3-642-23001-1
Volume 10:	Open Total Mesorectal Excision for Rectal Cancer	ISBN 978-3-642-23883-3
Volume 11:	Laparoscopic Sleeve Gastrectomy	ISBN 978-3-642-23889-5
Volume 12:	Laparoscopic Hysterectomy	ISBN 978-3-642-38093-8
Volume 13:	Video-assisted Thoracoscopic Lobectomy	ISBN 978-3-642-38543-8

Titles in preparation

Knotting and Tying
Anastomosis Techniques

NOTES

Printing: Ten Brink, Meppel, The Netherlands
Binding: Ten Brink, Meppel, The Netherlands